Biology of
Anxiety Disorders

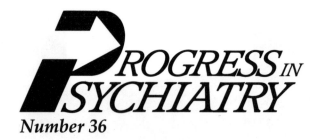

Number 36

David Spiegel, M.D.
Series Editor

Biology of Anxiety Disorders

Edited by
Rudolf Hoehn-Saric, M.D.
Daniel R. McLeod, Ph.D.

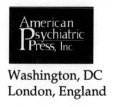
American Psychiatric Press, Inc.

Washington, DC
London, England

Copyright © 1993 American Psychiatric Press, Inc.
ALL RIGHTS RESERVED
Manufactured in the United States of America on acid-free paper
First Edition   96 95 94 93   4 3 2 1

American Psychiatric Press, Inc.
1400 K Street, N.W., Washington, DC   20005

Library of Congress Cataloging-in-Publication Data

Biology of anxiety disorders /   edited by Rudolf Hoehn-Saric, Daniel R. McLeod. — 1st ed.
    p.   cm. — (Progress in psychiatry series : 36)
Includes bibliographical references and index.
ISBN 0-88048-476-4 (alk. paper)
1. Anxiety—Physiological aspects.   I. Hoehn-Saric, Rudolf.
II.   McLeod, Daniel R.   III. Series.
  [DNLM: 1. Anxiety Disorders—physiopathology.   W1 PR6781L
  no. 36 /   WM 172 B615]
RC531.B473 1993
616.85'223—dc20
DNLM/DLC   92-17631
for Library of Congress   CIP

British Library Cataloguing in Publication Data

A CIP record is available from the British Library.

Contents

Contributors   vii

Introduction to the Progress in Psychiatry Series   ix
  David Spiegel, M.D.

Introduction   xv
  Rudolf Hoehn-Saric, M.D., and
  Daniel R. McLeod, Ph.D.

1 Cerebral Blood Flow and Metabolism
  in Anxiety Disorders   1
  William H. Wilson, Ph.D., and
  Roy J. Mathew, M.D.

2 Serotonin in the Pathogenesis of Anxiety   61
  René S. Kahn, M.D., and Clare Moore, M.S.

3 The Role of Corticotropin-Releasing Factor in the   103
  Pathophysiology of Anxiety Disorders
  Catherine Pihoker, M.D., and
  Charles B. Nemeroff, M.D., Ph.D.

4 Implications of Cocaine Kindling, Induction of the   121
  Proto-oncogene *c-fos*, and Contingent Tolerance
  in Panic Disorder
  R. M. Post, M.D., S. R. B. Weiss, Ph.D.,
  T. W. Uhde, M.D., M. Clark, Ph.D., and
  J. B. Rosen, Ph.D.

5 Somatic Manifestations of Normal and   177
  Pathological Anxiety
  Rudolf Hoehn-Saric, M.D., amd
  Daniel R. McLeod, Ph.D.

6 Perception of Physiological Changes in Normal   223
      and Pathological Anxiety
         Daniel R. McLeod, Ph.D., and
         Rudolf Hoehn-Saric, M.D.

7 Concluding Remarks   245
         Rudolf Hoehn-Saric, M.D., and
         Daniel R. McLeod, Ph.D.

     Index   251

Contributors

M. Clark, Ph.D.
Staff Fellow, Unit on Neurochemistry, Biological Psychiatry Branch, National Institute of Mental Health, Bethesda, Maryland

Rudolf Hoehn-Saric, M.D.
Professor of Psychiatry, Johns Hopkins School of Medicine, Johns Hopkins Hospital, Baltimore, Maryland

René S. Kahn, M.D.
Acting Unit Chief, Special Treatment Unit, Bronx Veterans Administration Hospital; Mount Sinai School of Medicine, New York, New York

Roy J. Mathew, M.D.
Professor of Psychiatry, Associate Professor of Radiology, Duke University Medical Center, Durham, North Carolina

Daniel R. McLeod, Ph.D.
Assistant Professor of Psychiatry, Johns Hopkins School of Medicine, Johns Hopkins Hospital, Baltimore, Maryland

Clare Moore, M.S.
Research Coordinator, Bronx Veterans Administration Hospital; Mount Sinai School of Medicine, New York, New York

Charles B. Nemeroff, M.D., Ph.D.
Professor and Chairman, Department of Psychiatry and Behavioral Sciences, Emory University School of Medicine, Atlanta, Georgia

Catherine Pihoker, M.D.
Assistant Professor of Pediatrics, University of Arkansas Medical School, Little Rock, Arkansas

R. M. Post, M.D.
Chief, Biological Psychiatry Branch, National Institute of Mental Health, Bethesda, Maryland

J. B. Rosen, Ph.D.
Staff Fellow, Unit on Neurochemistry, Biological Psychiatry Branch, National Institute of Mental Health, Bethesda, Maryland

T. W. Uhde, M.D.
Chief, Section on Anxiety and Affective Disorder, Biological Psychiatry Branch, National Institute of Mental Health, Bethesda, Maryland

S. R. B. Weiss, Ph.D.
Senior Staff Fellow, Biological Psychiatry Branch, National Institute of Mental Health, Bethesda, Maryland

William H. Wilson, Ph.D.
Associate Professor of Psychiatry, Division of Medical Psychology, Duke University Medical Center, Durham, North Carolina

Introduction to the Progress in Psychiatry Series

The Progress in Psychiatry Series is designed to capture in print the excitement that comes from assembling a diverse group of experts from various locations to examine in detail the newest information about a developing aspect of psychiatry. This series emerged as a collaboration between the American Psychiatric Association's (APA) Scientific Program Committee and the American Psychiatric Press, Inc. Great interest is generated by a number of the symposia presented each year at the APA annual meeting, and we realized that much of the information presented there, carefully assembled by people who are deeply immersed in a given area, would unfortunately not appear together in print. The symposia sessions at the annual meetings provide an unusual opportunity for experts who otherwise might not meet on the same platform to share their diverse viewpoints for a period of 3 hours. Some new themes are repeatedly reinforced and gain credence, while in other instances disagreements emerge, enabling the audience and now the reader to reach informed decisions about new directions in the field. The Progress in Psychiatry Series allows us to publish and capture some of the best of the symposia and thus provide an in-depth treatment of specific areas that might not otherwise be presented in broader review formats.

Psychiatry is by nature an interface discipline, combining the study of mind and brain, of individual and social environments, of the humane and the scientific. Thus, progress in the field is rarely linear—it often comes from unexpected sources. Further, new developments emerge from an array of viewpoints that do not necessarily provide immediate agreement but rather expert examination of the issues. We intend to present innovative ideas that will enable you, the reader, to participate in this process.

We believe the Progress in Psychiatry Series will provide you with an opportunity to review timely new information in specific fields of interest as they are developing. We hope you find that the excitement of the presentations is captured in the written word and that this book proves to be informative and enjoyable reading.

David Spiegel, M.D.
Series Editor
Progress in Psychiatry Series

Progress in Psychiatry Series Titles

The Borderline: Current Empirical Research (#1)
Edited by Thomas H. McGlashan, M.D.

Premenstrual Syndrome: Current Findings and Future Directions (#2)
Edited by Howard J. Osofsky, M.D., Ph.D., and Susan J. Blumenthal, M.D.

Treatment of Affective Disorders in the Elderly (#3)
Edited by Charles A. Shamoian, M.D.

Post-Traumatic Stress Disorder in Children (#4)
Edited by Spencer Eth, M.D., and Robert S. Pynoos, M.D., M.P.H.

The Psychiatric Implications of Menstruation (#5)
Edited by Judith H. Gold, M.D., F.R.C.P.C.

Can Schizophrenia Be Localized in the Brain? (#6)
Edited by Nancy C. Andreasen, M.D., Ph.D.

Medical Mimics of Psychiatric Disorders (#7)
Edited by Irl Extein, M.D., and Mark S. Gold, M.D.

Biopsychosocial Aspects of Bereavement (#8)
Edited by Sidney Zisook, M.D.

Psychiatric Pharmacosciences of Children and Adolescents (#9)
Edited by Charles Popper, M.D.

Psychobiology of Bulimia (#10)
Edited by James I. Hudson, M.D., and Harrison G. Pope, Jr., M.D.

Cerebral Hemisphere Function in Depression (#11)
Edited by Marcel Kinsbourne, M.D.

Eating Behavior in Eating Disorders (#12)
Edited by B. Timothy Walsh, M.D.

Tardive Dyskinesia: Biological Mechanisms and Clinical Aspects (#13)
Edited by Marion E. Wolf, M.D., and Aron D. Mosnaim, Ph.D.

Current Approaches to the Prediction of Violence (#14)
Edited by David A. Brizer, M.D., and Martha L. Crowner, M.D.

Treatment of Tricyclic-Resistant Depression (#15)
Edited by Irl L. Extein, M.D.

Depressive Disorders and Immunity (#16)
Edited by Andrew H. Miller, M.D.

Depression and Families: Impact and Treatment (#17)
Edited by Gabor I. Keitner, M.D.

Depression in Schizophrenia (#18)
Edited by Lynn E. DeLisi, M.D.

Biological Assessment and Treatment of Posttraumatic Stress Disorder (#19)
Edited by Earl L. Giller, Jr., M.D., Ph.D.

Personality Disorders: New Perspectives on Diagnostic Validity (#20)
Edited by John M. Oldham, M.D.

Serotonin in Major Psychiatric Disorders (#21)
Edited by Emil F. Coccaro, M.D., and Dennis L. Murphy, M.D.

Amino Acids in Psychiatric Disease (#22)
Edited by Mary Ann Richardson, Ph.D.

Family Environment and Borderline Personality Disorder (#23)
Edited by Paul Skevington Links, M.D.

Biological Rhythms, Mood Disorders, Light Therapy, and the Pineal Gland (#24)
Edited by Mohammad Shafii, M.D.,
and Sharon Lee Shafii, R.N., B.S.N.

Treatment Strategies for Refractory Depression (#25)
Edited by Steven P. Roose, M.D.,
and Alexander H. Glassman, M.D.

**Combination Pharmacotherapy and Psychotherapy
for Depression (#26)**
Edited by Donna Manning, M.D., and Allen J. Frances, M.D.

**The Neuroleptic Nonresponsive Patient: Characterization
and Treatment (#27)**
Edited by Burt Angrist, M.D., and S. Charles Schulz, M.D.

**Negative Schizophrenic Symptoms: Pathophysiology
and Clinical Implications (#28)**
Edited by John F. Greden, M.D., and Rajiv Tandon, M.D.

Neuropeptides and Psychiatric Disorders (#29)
Edited by Charles B. Nemeroff, M.D., Ph.D.

**Central Nervous System Peptide Mechanisms
in Stress and Depression (#30)**
Edited by S. Craig Risch, M.D.

**Current Concepts of Somatization: Research and Clinical
Perspectives (#31)**
Edited by Laurence J. Kirmayer, M.D., F.R.C.P.C.,
and James M. Robbins, Ph.D.

Mental Retardation: Developing Pharmacotherapies (#32)
Edited by John J. Ratey, M.D.

**Positron-Emission Tomography in Schizophrenia
Research (#33)**
Edited by Nora D. Volkow, M.D., and Alfred P. Wolf, Ph.D.

Brain Imaging in Affective Disorders (#34)
Edited by Peter Hauser, M.D.

Psychoimmunology Update (#35)
Edited by Jack M. Gorman, M.D., and Robert M. Kertzner, M.D.

Biology of Anxiety Disorders (#36)
Edited by Rudolf Hoehn-Saric, M.D.,
and Daniel R. McLeod, Ph.D.

Multiple Sclerosis: A Neuropsychiatric Disorder (#37)
Uriel Halbreich, M.D.

The Clinical Science of Electroconvulsive Therapy (#38)
C. Edward Coffey, M.D.

Psychopharmacology and Psychobiology of Ethnicity (#39)
Edited by Keh-Ming Lin, M.D., M.P.H., Russell E. Poland, Ph.D.,
and Gayle Nakasaki, M.S.W.

**Chronic Fatigue and Related Immune Deficiency
Syndromes (#40)**
Edited by Paul J. Goodnick, M.D., and Nancy G. Klimas, M.D.

Introduction

Anxiety is a universal experience. Under normal circumstances it functions as a biological warning system that enables a person to anticipate and often avoid potential harm or failure. Anxiety becomes abnormal when it is excessive in severity and duration, occurs in situations known to be harmless, or emerges spontaneously without apparent provocation.

Psychological aspects of anxiety have been studied over many decades. Recent advances in the physiology and pharmacology of the central nervous system, and technical advances, particularly in imaging, have opened new and exciting avenues toward a better understanding of the biology of anxiety. One advantage that anxiety research has over that of other psychiatric disorders is that animal models of anxiety are more plausible than those of other psychiatric disorders. This permits greater in-depth explorations of anxiety-related phenomena.

In this book recent advances in the biology of anxiety are reviewed. Out of necessity, areas of research that have been described in detail elsewhere and research whose significance is still unclear are omitted.

In Chapter 1, Wilson and Mathew review neuroimaging studies of anxiety. They discuss methods of imaging, the advantages and disadvantages of these procedures, and problems in interpretation. The authors also summarize the present literature, including their own extensive work.

Various neurotransmitters are associated with the biology of anxiety, of which the GABAergic system (Hommer et al. 1987) and the noradrenergic system (Gorman et al. 1989) have been most extensively explored. Other systems, such as the dopaminergic system (Antelman et al. 1988) and those systems involving histamine, opiate, adenosine (Hoehn-Saric 1982), and, more recently, cholecystokinin (Ravard and Dourish 1990), have also been found to be associated with the anxiety response. However, the roles of these neurotransmitters in anxiety still are poorly understood. The serotonergic system has for a long time been thought to be associated with anxiety, but conflicting data from animal studies, as well as the absence of drugs that specifically alter the serotonergic system, have impeded research on serotonin, which has thus taken a back seat to research on the noradrenergic system. Recent pharmacological advances, described by Kahn and Moore in Chapter 2, however, show that the serotonergic system may be as important as the noradrenergic system in the biology of anxiety. The serotonergic system also appears to play a role in the regulation of psychic anxiety and obsessive-compulsive symptoms, perhaps by modifying the function of the frontal lobes (Hoehn-Saric et al. 1991a).

In Chapter 3, Pihoker and Nemeroff describe the role of corticotropin-releasing factor (CRF) in anxiety. The discovery of the role of CRF in stress, anxiety, and depression has been of exceeding importance because disturbances in CRF may constitute the biological link between the frequently coexisting conditions of anxiety and depression.

The work of Post and colleagues, in Chapter 4, illustrates how basic research and clinical observations complement each other. Kindling in the limbic system leads to long-term changes that may be important in the genesis of seizures and possibly in recurrent depression and paroxysmal anxiety disorders, such as panic disorder. Moreover, kindling appears to be the pathological extension of long-term potentiation, a neurobiological process that is associated with learning and memory. The phenomena described in this chapter may be related to changes associated not only with panic attacks but also with the acquisition of a fear response, such as agoraphobia in panic disorder, or situational fear in social phobia (Hoehn-Saric et al. 1991b).

Anxiety manifests itself not only in the brain but in the entire body as well. In Chapter 5, Hoehn-Saric and McLeod review peripheral physiological manifestations of normal and abnormal anxiety. The authors discuss how normal anxiety differs from pathological anxiety and show how the various anxiety disorders differ quantitatively as well as qualitatively in their physiological expression.

Patients vary greatly in how they perceive peripheral manifestations of anxiety. Ultimately, it is the brain that receives and interprets changes that occur in the body. In Chapter 6, McLeod and Hoehn-Saric review the relationship between objective bodily changes during anxiety and the subjective perception of these changes. The authors offer several explanations for the frequently observed discrepancies between physiological changes and their perception. With this chapter, followed by some concluding remarks in Chapter 7, the authors close a loop: anxiety, generated in the brain, affects the entire body, which in turn sends signals back to the brain, which then interprets all of the information, producing an affective-cognitive experience.

Rudolf Hoehn-Saric, M.D.
Daniel R. McLeod, Ph.D.

REFERENCES

Antelman SM, Knopf S, Caggiula AR, et al: Stress and enhanced dopamine utilization in the frontal cortex: the myth and the reality, in The Mesocorticolimbic Dopamine System. Ann N Y Acad Sci 537:273–291, 1988

Gorman JM, Liebowitz MR, Fyer AJ, et al: A neuroanatomical hypothesis for panic disorder. Am J Psychiatry 146:148–161, 1989

Hoehn-Saric R: Neurotransmitters in anxiety. Arch Gen Psychiatry 39:735–742, 1982

Hoehn-Saric R, Harris GJ, Pearlson GD, et al: A fluoxetine-induced frontal lobe syndrome in an obsessive-compulsive patient. J Clin Psychiatry 52:131–133, 1991a

Hoehn-Saric R, McLeod DR, Glowa JR: The effects of NMDA receptor blockade on the acquisition of a conditioned emotional response. Biol Psychiatry 30:170–176, 1991b

Hommer DW, Skolnick P, Paul SM: The benzodiazepine/GABA receptor complex and anxiety, in Psychopharmacology: The Third Generation of Progress. Edited by Meltzer HY. New York, Raven, 1987, pp 977–983

Ravard S, Dourish CT: Cholecystokinin and anxiety. Trends in Pharmacological Sciences 11:271–273, 1990

Chapter 1

Cerebral Blood Flow and Metabolism in Anxiety Disorders

William H. Wilson, Ph.D., and Roy J. Mathew, M.D.

A variety of physiological changes are known to be associated with anxiety disorders. Both general circulation and blood flow to specific vascular beds are usually affected. Although brain blood flow and metabolism are of considerable clinical significance, the effects of anxiety on these physiological manifestations of brain function have only recently come under extensive study as less invasive techniques have become available. In this chapter we review the ways in which anxiety might influence cerebral blood flow (CBF) and cerebral metabolic rate (CMR) and describe the results of studies on this topic. Possible clinical implications of anxiety-related CBF and CMR changes are discussed.

NEUROPHYSIOLOGY OF AROUSAL AND ANXIETY

The Brain-Stem Reticular Formation

The concept of arousal is central to the neurophysiology of anxiety. Arousal refers to levels of generalized, diffuse activation of the brain. The concept is supported by electroencephalographic and neurophysiological experiments and physiological studies of

The work represented in this chapter was supported in part by National Institute of Mental Health Grant MH-42232.

1

"behavioral energetics" (Duffy 1972; Lader 1982; Malmo 1959). One of the first regions to be clearly associated with arousal was the *brain-stem reticular formation* (Moruzzi and Magoun 1949). The brain-stem reticular formation was originally thought to be diffuse and nonspecific, but more recent studies have identified ascending and descending pathways, facilitatory and inhibitory components, and functionally specialized groups of neurons (based on their anatomic location and chemical characteristics) within the network of reticular neurons (Kandel and Schwartz 1981; Siegel 1979). Such groups of reticular neurons, such as the norepinephrine-containing locus coeruleus and the serotonin-containing raphe nuclei, are well known for their neuropsychiatric significance. Although these neuron groupings have been ascribed other functions, there is general agreement that the brain-stem reticular core is intimately related to arousal.

The Limbic System

Evidence suggesting the involvement of other brain regions in arousal is more complex and less well established. The limbic system, to which the reticular formation is connected, is hypothesized to have a role in autonomic activity and arousal. Having both facilitatory and inhibitory components and involvement in several physiological functions (i.e., hunger, thirst, sex drive, aggression, memory), this system would seem to be related to arousal. An extensive body of information is available on the anatomy and physiology of the limbic system (Isaacson 1982). Several complex arousal systems that incorporate the reticular formation and limbic system have been postulated (Fowles 1980; Routtenberg 1968).

The Cerebral Cortex

The nature of involvement of the cerebral cortex in arousal would seem less controversial. The frontal lobes have been identified as the cortical region having the most intimate connections with parts of the subcortical arousal system including the thalamus and upper parts of the brain stem. The frontal lobes also have dense connections with other cortical regions (Kelly 1976; Nauta 1971). Thus, it would seem highly likely that the frontal lobes constitute the cortical apparatus responsible for maintaining levels of activation of the brain. This possibility is supported by a large body of clinical and experimental evidence, especially those findings provided by Luria and colleagues (Fuster 1980; Luria 1973; Pribram 1973). The well-known electroencephalographic pattern of predominantly higher-frequency waveforms over the frontal lobe during wakefulness supports this hypothesis. It should also be noted that the cortical gray matter is thicker on cross-section over the frontal regions compared with that over the occipital pole (Carpenter 1976; Noback 1975). In addition to arousal, more complicated functions closely related to wakefulness, such as abstract thought, synthetic reasoning, and organization of independent behaviors in time and space toward future goals, have also been ascribed to the frontal lobes (Goldman-Rakic 1984).

The temporal poles may have a specific role in anxiety and arousal. Based on animal studies, they have been hypothesized to be involved in the interpretation of environmental information (Mesulam and Mufson 1982; Moran et al. 1987). As human studies have shown, fear and anxiety are often associated with temporal lobe pathology such as epilepsy (Gloor et al. 1982; Halgren and Walter 1978) and may develop after removal of the temporal lobe (Wall et al. 1986). Fontaine et al. (1987) have reported the results of magnetic resonance imaging (MRI) scans of 13 patients with panic disorder, of whom 54% had some abnormalities and 5 of 13 had abnormalities in the white matter of the temporal lobe and on the right, whereas none of the control subjects had these changes.

A growing body of literature suggests hemispheric differences in the mediation of emotions, and a greater role has been ascribed to the right hemisphere (Galin 1974; Prohovnik 1978; Ross 1984). This may, however, be an oversimplification in the case of anxiety. Studies conducted by Tucker and associates (1977) indicate that differing levels of anxiety may be associated with asymmetrical hemispheric activation and performance. Mild situational stress was found to be associated with greater right hemispheric contribution to cognition (Tucker et al. 1977). However, later studies involving highly anxious subjects showed an excessive reliance on left-hemispheric cognitive processing (Tucker et al.

1978; Tyler and Tucker 1982). Because the few studies conducted in this area relied on indirect techniques for assessing brain function, no firm conclusions are warranted.

MEASUREMENT TECHNIQUES AND ISSUES

In the normal brain, CBF and CMR are closely related to brain function (Raichle et al. 1976), and the former two have been used as indices of the latter in psychiatric research (Mathew et al. 1985a). A comparative description of measurement techniques is presented in Table 1–1.

Among the first CBF methods used in psychiatric research was the *nitrous oxide inhalation technique* (the first *quantitative* CBF measurement technique) developed by Kety and Schmidt (1948). This technique, which yielded only a single value for the entire brain, was followed by the *intracarotid injection technique* (Ingvar and Lassen 1961), which involved injecting xenon-133 (^{133}Xe) into the internal carotid artery and monitoring the progressive decline in radioactivity over the scalp with a system of scintillation detectors. CBF was calculated from these scalp clearance curves. Obrist and associates (1975) developed a totally noninvasive CBF measurement technique in which intracarotid injection was replaced by ^{133}Xe inhalation. The intracarotid and inhalation xenon techniques measure only blood flow to the cerebral cortex from where most of the measured radioactivity originated, and are thus considered two-dimensional techniques. Development of three-dimensional tomographic techniques such as single-photon emission computed tomography (SPECT) (Price et al. 1980) and positron-emission tomography (PET) (Mazziotta 1985) has made both cortical and subcortical CBF, as well as CMR, measurement possible.

There are similarities and many differences among two-dimensional and three-dimensional measurement techniques. Both two- and three-dimensional techniques are based on the rate of accumulation and/or clearance of radioactive tracers by the brain. In two-dimensional techniques, the rate of clearance is estimated by recording the progressive decline of radioactivity using stationary scintillation detectors applied to the scalp. The detectors register radiation mostly from the superficial parts of

Table 1-1. Techniques for the measurement of cerebral blood flow (CBF) and cerebral metabolic rate (CMR)

Technique	Invasiveness	Irradiation	CBF/CMR	Bilateral/ unilateral	Carotid/ vertebrobasilar	Spatial resolution
Nitrous oxide inhalation	Arterial and internal jugular puncture	Absent	CBF and CMR	Ipsilateral hemisphere only	Both	A single value for the entire hemisphere
Intracarotid ^{133}Xe injection	Carotid puncture	0.5 mrad (gonads)	CBF	Ipsilateral hemisphere only	Carotid vascular bed only	1 cm
^{133}Xe inhalation	Venous puncture	2.9 mrad (gonads) 102 mrad (lung)	CBF	Both hemispheres	Both carotid and vertebrobasilar beds	3–4 cm
SPECT[a] (^{133}Xe)	Venous puncture	5.0 mrad (gonads) 360 mrad (lung)	CBF	Both hemispheres	Both carotid and vertebrobasilar beds	1.7 cm
PET[b] [^{18}F]FDG[c]	Arterial puncture	63 mrad/mCi (gonads) 43 mrad/mCi (total body)	CBF and CMR	Both hemispheres	Both carotid and vertebrobasilar beds	0.7–1.7 cm

[a]Single-photon emission computed tomography.
[b]Positron-emission tomography.
[c]^{18}F-labeled fluorodeoxyglucose.

the brain (cortex) because the tracer used (^{133}Xe) is a low gamma energy emitter (81 KeV) (Sakai et al. 1979). The scalp scintillation detectors will not "see" blood flow to deeper brain structures and the medial part of the hemispheres.

Three-dimensional techniques such as PET utilize positron-emitting tracers that produce higher gamma energy photons (e.g., 511 KeV [1,000 electron volts] in PET) from annihilation reactions. There are several positron-emitting tracers that have been used, including ^{15}O, ^{13}N, ^{11}C, ^{18}F, and ^{77}Kr. A freely diffusible, very short–half-life tracer such as ^{15}O-labeled water is commonly used to quantify blood flow, while ^{11}C-labeled glucose or a metabolically inert analog such as ^{18}F-labeled fluorodeoxyglucose (FDG) is used to measure cerebral metabolism of glucose. Tomographic slices of the brain are taken with gamma cameras or rotating gantries of scintillation detectors (Powers and Raichle 1986). To convert the count rates into CBF or CMR values it is necessary to employ *tracer-kinetic models*, which are mathematical models of how the tracer behaves, and to take into consideration a number of variables such as half-life and rate of delivery to the brain (Reiman 1990). Thus, the nature of information provided by the two- versus three-dimensional techniques varies substantially, and both approaches have advantages and disadvantages.

Problems associated with the two-dimensional techniques include such factors as lower spatial resolution, contamination of scalp radioactivity by isotope trapped in frontal sinuses, and overlapping of the cortical and subcortical flows (the "look-through" effect). To some extent these latter two problems are dealt with effectively by the mathematical model used to determine blood flow. Two-dimensional techniques separate gray matter and white matter flow by using a bicompartmental model (Obrist et al. 1975) in clearance-curve analysis based on the well-established fact that gray matter perfusion is three to four times higher than white matter flow. The xenon inhalation technique is noninvasive, and, because of the low level of radiation of ^{133}Xe, many repeated measurements may be made before reaching the yearly dosing limit established by the U.S. Food and Drug Administration. The inhalation technique has been shown to be reliable in repeated-measures studies (Blauenstein et al. 1977).

Problems associated with the three-dimensional techniques include much higher levels of radiation exposure (thus limiting the total number of scans that can be done in a year for safety reasons), the need for multiple arterial blood samples to determine absolute CBF and CMR, and, not least, the considerably higher cost. For the CMR glucose technique using the ^{18}F-labeled FDG method, a considerable time must be allowed to elapse (e.g., 24 hours) between measurements so that the tracer can clear, because the normal metabolic path of glucose cannot process deoxyglucose and the end product (i.e., deoxyglucose-6-phosphate) is trapped in the cerebral tissue (Frackowiak 1986). Barlett and associates (1988) have shown in a test-retest reliability study that resting glucose metabolic rates have a low intrasubject variability and high stability over a 24-hour period. Three-dimensional (i.e., tomographic) techniques depend upon their spatial resolution to separate gray and white matter flows. Cortical gray matter, while large in surface area, is relatively thin in tomographic slices (2–5 mm) (Guyton 1987). The three-dimensional techniques have a much better spatial resolution as compared with the two-dimensional ones, but it is still well above 5 mm. The problem of imaging cortex satisfactorily on tomographic images is further complicated by technical difficulties in separating cerebrospinal fluid and white matter (low radioactivity area) from the undulated cortical gray (high radioactivity areas) (i.e., a partial volume artifact, which is when the area being measured is smaller than the sensitivity of the instrument) (Powers and Raichle 1986).

HYPERFRONTALITY

One of the areas of difference between two- and three-dimensional techniques involves the concept of *hyperfrontality*. Ingvar first described an anterior-posterior difference in CBF, reporting a 20% to 40% difference in blood flow to the frontal regions under resting conditions. He ascribed this difference to the role played by the frontal lobes in maintaining wakefulness (Ingvar 1979), in addition to complicated functions (Goldman-Rakic 1984). The concept of increased frontal activity during wakefulness is supported by a wide body of clinical and experimental evidence. The frontal lobes are known to have dense connections with subcortical regions that are believed to mediate "nonspecific arousal" (Kelly 1976; Nauta 1971; Stuss and Benson 1986). A wide range of neurophysiological and neuropsychological studies point to the association between arousal and the frontal lobes. The frontal lobes are also involved in sensory data processing, cognition, volition, and initiation of motor activity (Fuster 1980; Luria 1973; Stuss and Benson 1986). The well-known electroencephalographic pattern of predominant waveforms of higher frequency over the frontal lobes during wakefulness provides additional support for the frontal lobes' role in maintaining arousal (Ingvar and Soderberg 1958; Menon et al. 1980).

The hyperfrontal pattern of CBF distribution becomes more pronounced when arousal is increased through stimulation (Ingvar and Lassen 1976; Risberg et al. 1977). Intravenous administration of nonsedating doses of diazepam, which is known to induce tranquilization, reduced frontal perfusion more significantly than it did flow to other parts of the brain (Mathew et al. 1985b). Slow-wave sleep attenuates the hyperfrontal pattern of CBF distribution (Townsend et al. 1973), and hyperfrontality is absent in comatose states (Deutsch and Eisenberg 1987). Thus, the available evidence adds validity to the finding of a hyperfrontal pattern of CBF distribution during wakefulness in normal subjects.

Increased frontal perfusion in normal subjects during wakefulness has been reported by all laboratories that utilized two-dimensional CBF measurement techniques (Blauenstein et al. 1977; Gur et al. 1985; Mamo et al. 1983; Mathew et al. 1986; Meyer et al. 1978; Prohovnik et al. 1980; Weinberger et al. 1986; Wilkinson et al. 1969). However, this finding has been inconsistently replicated by the majority of laboratories that utilized three-dimensional CBF and CMR measurement techniques (Devous et al. 1986; Rapoport et al. 1985). Buchsbaum and associates (1982) have consistently reported higher glucose metabolism (measured with PET) in the frontal gray matter as compared with that found in the posterior brain regions. Metter and colleagues (1984) found only partial support for hyperfrontality with PET scan measurements of glucose metabolism; the frontal value was higher only when the superior frontal region was compared with the posterior temporal regions; the occipital and Wernicke's regions had values that were on the average higher than the frontal measures. Similar findings were reported by Meyer et al. (1981), who measured CBF with another three-dimensional technique, computed tomography (CT) scanning, during stable xenon inhalation. Devous and co-workers (1986) could not find hyperfrontality in their study using the three-dimensional technique SPECT (with ^{133}Xe).

Cerebral blood flow changes, such as hyperfrontality, that are believed to be related to arousal are of considerable relevance to the study of anxiety. Thus, the inconsistent replication of the findings of hyperfrontality with two-dimensional measurement techniques by more recent three-dimensional techniques needs to be examined closely.

A number of factors have been considered to explain the difference (Mathew 1989). Contamination of the frontal flow values measured with the two-dimensional techniques by the isotope trapped in the frontal sinuses has been offered as an explanation for hyperfrontality (Devous et al. 1986). This would, however, seem to be inadequate because hyperfrontality is most obvious over the superior frontal areas—that is, away from the frontal sinuses—in most subjects. [133]Xe is the tracer used for all currently available two-dimensional CBF techniques, and it is possible that the blood-brain partition coefficient for xenon is higher over the frontal lobe as compared with the rest of the brain. However, it should be noted that hyperfrontality could not be detected by CBF measurements with three-dimensional techniques (SPECT) using ^{133}Xe as a tracer (Devous et al. 1986).

Differences between the two types of techniques in the accuracy of gray matter measurements constitute another possible explanation. As noted above, cortical gray matter, while large in surface area, is relatively thin on cross-section; in most regions it is much less than 5 mm (Carpenter 1976). The three-dimensional techniques used for CBF measurement have a spatial resolution above 5 mm. The problem is made worse by the partial volume artifact (i.e., when the area being measured is smaller than the sensitivity of the instrument) created by technical difficulties in separating cerebrospinal fluid and white matter (low radioactivity area) from the undulating cortical gray (high radioactivity areas) (Powers and Raichle 1986). For two-dimensional techniques, on the other hand, the separation is made by the analysis of the scalp clearance curves (Obrist et al. 1975). As yet there is no satisfactory answer for this problem.

Availability of these sophisticated measurement techniques has made research on psychiatric disorders less difficult. Indeed, large numbers of CBF and CMR studies have been carried out on patients with different psychiatric disorders, including anxiety disorders. These research projects have yielded meaningful information on abnormal brain function in psychiatric disorders, but they also have uncovered some difficulties in this line of research. Although CBF and brain function are closely coupled, CBF (especially global flow) is influenced by other factors such as the autonomic nervous system, blood viscosity, and carbon dioxide levels, among others (Mathew et al. 1986).

RELATIONSHIP OF ANXIETY
TO AROUSAL

The majority of psychophysiological studies support the hypothesis that anxiety is a hyperarousal state (Duffy 1972; Lader 1975). For example, electroencephalography, which probably is a direct measure of arousal, shows fairly consistent and predictable changes in anxiety—that is, less alpha and more beta frequency than normal. Peripheral physiological changes, mostly involving the autonomic nervous system, also show evidence of overactivity. However, it should be noted that these changes occur as well in such emotional states as anger and excitement (Duffy 1972). Anxiety and these emotions have been hypothesized to have the same physiological substrate (i.e., increased arousal). The precise nature of the emotion depends upon the subject's perception and interpretation of the environment (Lader 1982; Sarason 1984; Schachter and Singer 1962). However, because the subjective experiences of these emotions are different, one would expect neurobiological differences among them. Even the peripheral neurophysiological factors that differentiate different emotions are controversial and poorly understood (Ax 1953), and very little is known about the associated brain mechanisms.

AROUSAL, CEREBRAL BLOOD FLOW, AND CEREBRAL METABOLIC RATE

Global Changes

It is generally recognized that, under normal conditions, cerebral function leads to an increase in metabolic demand that then is closely supported by an increase in blood flow. Therefore, regional differences in function should in turn be reflected in regional differences in CMR and thus CBF (Mazziotta 1985; Raichle et al. 1976). Changes in level of arousal should be associated with parallel changes in CBF and CMR. Conditions characterized by increase in arousal, such as REM sleep, mental activation, and epileptic seizures, are indeed associated with CBF increases (Broderson et al. 1973; Gur et al. 1982; Meyer et al. 1978; Risberg et al. 1981; Sakai et al. 1980; Townsend et al. 1973), and conditions characterized by hypoarousal, such as drug-induced narcosis, slow-wave sleep, and coma, are associated with global decreases in CBF (Forster et al. 1982; Frewen et al. 1985; Obrist et al. 1979; Rockoff et al. 1980; Vernheit et al. 1978). Additional support for the association between global CBF and arousal is provided by the close relationship between the electroencephalogram (EEG) (which has been extensively utilized in arousal research) and CBF (Ingvar and Soderberg 1956; Menon et al. 1980).

Similar findings with CMR have been reported utilizing PET methodology. For example, studies of glucose metabolism by Mazziotta and associates (1981, 1982) in normal volunteers have shown that although there is a left-right symmetry at rest, there is a progressive decline in CMR with sensory deprivation (eyes and/or ears occluded), with greater decreases in the right hemisphere and regional differences (i.e., greatest left-right differences in parts of the frontal, temporal, and occipital cortex). In studies with sleeping subjects, Heiss et al. (1985) have noted a general decrease in CMR during slow-wave sleep but an increase in activity during dreaming. These results with humans are consistent with findings reported from studies on primates (e.g., Kennedy et al. 1982).

Brain Stem

Two lines of evidence support an association between global CBF and levels of activity within the brain stem, which, as was pointed out earlier, is believed to mediate arousal. Juge and associates (1979) demonstrated correlations between blood flow to the brain stem and cerebellar regions, and state of awareness as judged by clinical and EEG evaluations in semi-coma, stupor, slow-wave sleep, drowsiness, rest, activation, REM sleep, and epileptic seizures. Ingvar and co-workers (1964) measured CBF with two different measurement techniques in a 60-year-old patient who was in a comatose state following an acute vascular lesion of the brain stem. Air encephalography revealed only moderate degrees of cerebral atrophy. The EEG showed severe depression with low-voltage slow waves. Cortical biopsy taken from the left frontal lobe showed normal findings, with no evidence of neuronal loss or gliosis. CBF and cerebral oxygen consumption were found to be significantly reduced. These findings would seem to suggest that the upper brain-stem lesion was responsible for the coma and the associated reduction in CBF and CMR. Ingvar and Soderberg (1958) also demonstrated cortical blood flow increase related to EEG patterns evoked by stimulation of the brain stem.

Frontal Cortex

Cerebral blood flow research also supports the involvement of the frontal lobe in the arousal mechanism. Ingvar (1979) first reported a 20% to 40% increase in blood flow to the frontal regions as compared with the occipital and temporal regions in 11 patients undergoing carotid angiography while awake but resting. The author ascribed this CBF increase to the activity of the frontal lobe in maintaining wakefulness. This "hyperfrontal" pattern of CBF distribution became more pronounced when arousal was increased through stimulation (Ingvar and Lassen 1976). During slow-wave sleep, the hyperfrontal pattern of flow distribution became less significant (Townsend et al. 1973).

Risberg and colleagues (1977) studied the CBF changes associated with the administration of a problem-solving test on two consecutive days. During the first test administration, both frontal and posterior flow increased. However, during the second test administration, only the posterior flow increased, while frontal flow remained the same. The frontal flow increase was attributed to the apprehension associated with the novelty of the test, which was absent during the second session. (In experiments involving repeated CBF measurements under resting conditions, the second set of values tend to be lower than the first. This also may be due to habituation to the measurement technique [Warach et al. 1987].) Therefore, degrees of hyperfrontality would seem to be related to degrees of brain activation, thus supporting the association between the frontal lobe and arousal. However, as was noted earlier, there are differences in results on hyperfrontality depending on the methodology employed, and these findings are not consistently replicated with the PET procedure.

Tranquilization and Cerebral Blood Flow

We conducted a study on the effect of nonsedating doses of diazepam, a commonly used tranquilizer, on regional CBF in normal human subjects (Mathew et al. 1985b). Twenty volunteers, free of significant medical and psychiatric disorders, participated in the project. Regional CBF was measured twice in each participant, at an interval of 30 minutes. Five minutes before the second measurement of CBF, one-half of the subjects, randomly determined, were given an intravenous injection of diazepam (0.1 mg/kg; mean = 7 mg, SD = 1.6 mg); the other 10 subjects (5 males and 5 females) were administered an intravenous injection of saline. The injections were given under double-blind conditions. The subjects were specifically instructed to stay awake and keep their eyes open, and they were questioned about levels of wakefulness during the postmeasurement debriefing. During the CBF measurements, respiratory rate, end-tidal CO_2 levels (PE_{CO_2}), and a one-channel EEG were continuously recorded. None of the subjects became drowsy during the experiment. The CBF values obtained during the second measurement for each participant were adjusted for differences in PE_{CO_2} (Maximilian et al. 1980).

Mathew et al.'s findings indicate that intravenous administration of small, nonsedating doses of diazepam was accompanied by a global reduction in CBF that was more marked in the right hemisphere, and especially in the frontal lobe. Milder CBF changes in the same direction were seen in the left hemisphere. These findings therefore support the hypothesis that the frontal lobe is involved in the mediation of levels of arousal. Thus, available data clearly support the positive relationship between CBF, CMR, and arousal; the measurement techniques are able to differentiate changes in local regions of interest under different states of arousal.

OTHER FACTORS INFLUENCING CEREBRAL BLOOD FLOW AND CEREBRAL METABOLIC RATE

Cerebral blood flow, CMR, and brain function are coupled, and both CBF and CMR have been used as indices of brain function in studies of arousal. Thus, these two indices would seem to be of use in identifying the neuroanatomic substrates of anxiety. Unfortunately, both indices can be influenced by factors other than brain function, and these factors need to be taken into account when designing studies and interpreting results. A list of variables that are known to have effects on CBF and CMR and the direction of those effects in normal subjects are given in Table 1–2. These variables must be considered in any study of anxiety

Table 1–2. Variables that may be important in studies of anxiety and their effects on brain blood flow and metabolism

Variables	CBF	CMR
Aging	Decrease	Decrease
Gender	M < F	M < F[a]
Hypercapnia	Increase	Increase[a]
Hypoxia	Increase	Increase[a]
Arousal level	Increase	Increase
Epinephrine	Increase	Increase
Norepinephrine	Decrease	No change

Note. CBF = cerebral blood flow; CMR = cerebral metabolism rate.
[a]Effects have been reported in the indicated direction; however, controversy exists about results.

disorders. As was pointed out earlier, anxiety is associated with a variety of physiological and biochemical changes, some of which may be relevant to the measurement of CBF and CMR and thus are issues to be considered.

Catecholamines

Stress and acute anxiety are very well known to increase epinephrine and norepinephrine in the periphery (Frankenhaeuser 1971; Levi 1972; Mathew et al. 1982a). The possible effects of these substances on brain blood flow can therefore be important. Intravenous epinephrine infusions have been found to increase CBF and CMR by over 200% in animals (Abdul-Rahman et al. 1979; Dahlgren et al. 1980). Gibbs and co-workers (1935) reported increased CBF following intravenous epinephrine infusion in human subjects. The authors measured CBF with a thermoelectric flow meter inserted in the internal jugular vein. Kety (1952) investigated the effect of epinephrine and norepinephrine infusions on CBF and cerebral oxygen consumption with the nitrous oxide inhalation technique. CBF and cerebral metabolism were calculated based on the arteriovenous differences in nitrous oxide, glucose, carbon dioxide, oxygen, and pyruvate. While norepinephrine infusions were not associated with any significant changes, epinephrine increased CBF by 21% and cerebral oxygen consumption by 22%. King and associates (1952), using the same measurement technique, showed that the increases in CBF and cerebral oxygen consumption following epinephrine infusion were not associated with changes in cerebrovascular resistance. This finding would seem to argue against the possibility of the increase in CBF being due to a direct vascular effect of epinephrine. Norepinephrine, on the other hand, was found to increase cerebrovascular resistance and reduce CBF. However, Sensenbach and associates (1953) could not replicate these findings. No changes in CBF, cerebrovascular resistance, or cerebral oxygen utilization were found following epinephrine injections; norepinephrine injections, on the other hand, reduced CBF.

Olesen and co-workers injected epinephrine and isoproterenol into the internal carotid artery in human subjects and measured CBF via the ^{133}Xe intracarotid injection technique (Olesen 1975;

Olesen et al. 1971). This technique, similar to the other two-dimensional techniques, measures cerebral blood flow to cortical gray matter only. Intracarotid isoproterenol and epinephrine were not, in fact, found to be associated with any changes in CBF.

In summary, in several animal experiments and human studies, investigators have found increases in CBF following intravenous epinephrine infusions. Intracarotid epinephrine and isoproterenol, on the other hand, do not affect CBF. Thus, in all probability, the epinephrine-induced CBF changes are secondary to the behavioral manifestations of the drugs and are not due to the drugs' direct vascular effects. The latter is important because adrenergic receptors (alpha and beta) have been demonstrated on cerebral microvasculature (Harik et al. 1981). Norepinephrine may reduce CBF, but it is unclear whether this reduction is due to the direct effect of the drug on cerebral blood vessels.

Recent years have seen an upsurge of interest in the central nervous system (CNS) biochemistry of anxiety. Evidence suggesting the involvement of such neurotransmitters as norepinephrine, serotonin, and gamma-aminobutyric acid (GABA) has been reported (Hoehn-Saric 1982). Large numbers of norepinephrine- and serotonin-containing neurons in the brain-stem centers have been shown to innervate cerebral capillaries (intraparenchymal innervation) and form varicosities from which neurotransmitters are released. These fibers have also been shown to make synaptic contacts with other neurons. An extensive body of literature is available on the effects of intravenous, intracarotid, and intraventricular infusions and cortical applications of these neurotransmitters on CBF. Cerebral blood vessels are also known to contain appreciable quantities of enzymes relevant to the synthesis and destruction of these neurotransmitters. These enzymes include tyrosine hydroxylase, monoamine oxidase, dopamine beta-hydroxylase, and tryptophan hydroxylase. The influence of these neurotransmitters on CBF is a complicated and controversial matter, and a detailed discussion of this is beyond the scope of this chapter. Interested readers should consult the review by Edvinsson and Mackenzie (1977). Much less is known about the influence of these substances on anxiety-related changes in CBF and CMR.

Autonomic Nervous System

Activation of the autonomic nervous system, especially the sympathetic division, is an integral part of acute anxiety. Sympathetic stimulation is believed to be responsible for anxiety-related circulatory changes in such peripheral vascular beds as the muscle and skin: anxiety increases blood flow to the muscle and decreases flow to the skin (Ackner 1956; Kelly and Walter 1969). Sympathetic fibers also innervate cerebral blood vessels in humans and other animals, and adrenergic receptors have been demonstrated on cerebral microvasculature (Busija and Heistad 1984a). Nerve fibers containing the neurotransmitters epinephrine and norepinephrine are present in the walls of pial and cerebral parenchymal capillaries. The sympathetic fibers originate from the ipsilateral superior cervical ganglion. Nerve endings on cerebral blood vessels contain considerable amounts of norepinephrine and have an active, specific uptake mechanism. Adrenergic agonists such as phentolamine and yohimbine release tritiated norepinephrine from brain blood vessels when preloaded with the labeled neurotransmitter, and this efflux is reduced by clonidine. For additional details, the reader should consult the review articles by Edvinsson and Mackenzie (1977), Edvinsson (1982), and Busija and Heistad (1984b).

Cerebral blood flow response to sympathetic stimulation varies across different species; in humans, a 5% to 15% reduction in CBF is seen (Edvinsson 1982). There is general consensus that brain blood vessels are less responsive to sympathetic stimulation in comparison with peripheral vessels. Thus, in normal subjects, the autonomic nervous system may have only an insignificant role in the control of CBF, even during anxiety. However, it is quite likely that the cerebral vasculature in anxious patients is much more sensitive to sympathetic activation than in normal subjects; patients with panic disorders have been shown to be oversensitive to sympathetic stimulation in the periphery (Nesse et al. 1984).

Hemorheology

An increase in hematocrit and blood viscosity secondary to stress has been referred to as *polycytosis* (Benitone and Kling 1970;

Dameshek 1953; Dintenfass and Zador 1976, 1977; Lawrence and Berlin 1951; Russell and Conley 1964; Wilson and Boyle 1952). Hematocrit in the range of 50% to 56% and hemoglobin levels between 16 and 18 grams percent are the commonly accepted criteria for this syndrome (Benitone and Kling 1970; Dameshek 1953). Blood viscosity is known to influence CBF: CBF is increased in conditions associated with low blood viscosity (i.e., anemia) and reduced in conditions associated with high blood viscosity (i.e., polycythemia) (Thomas 1982). There is some uncertainty as to whether this inverse relationship between blood viscosity and CBF depends on alterations in blood rheology or on the associated changes in oxygen delivery to the brain (Marshall 1982).

Anxiety-related changes in blood viscosity can thus be very important to CBF. However, careful examination of the literature on stress polycytosis shows that none of the studies established a positive association between stress and increased blood viscosity. Most investigators measured hematocrit in subjects with vague symptoms of anxiety, in patients referred to hematology clinics with elevated hematocrit for which no other explanations could be found, in patients with a wide variety of ill-defined psychiatric disorders, or in patients with hypertension. Few investigators used standard criteria for making psychiatric diagnosis, and no attempt was made to correlate degrees of distress, anxiety, or depression with the hematocrit elevations. Stress polycytosis is believed to be more common in males than in females (Dameshek 1953; Russell and Conley 1964). Hematocrit is normally higher in males (Kelly and Munan 1977). However, the assumption that males may be more stressed than females is questionable in view of the higher incidence of anxiety and depression in the latter.

To study the relationship between stress and polycytosis, we examined the possibility of an anxiety-related increase in hematocrit in a group of patients with a DSM-III (American Psychiatric Association 1980) diagnosis of generalized anxiety disorder (GAD) (Mathew and Wilson 1986). All participants were physically healthy and medication free for a minimum of 2 weeks prior to the study. Blood samples were drawn twice: 3 minutes and then 10 minutes after venipuncture. During these 10 minutes, 12 patients received an intravenous infusion of epinephrine (0.2

µg/kg/min), while the remaining 12 patients received saline infusions. There were 6 males and 6 females in both groups of patients. The patients were assigned to the epinephrine and saline groups on a random basis, and the infusions were given under double-blind conditions. Measurements of pulse rate and blood pressure were taken before each blood sample, and levels of anxiety at the time of blood sample withdrawal were quantified with the State Anxiety Scale of the State-Trait Anxiety Inventory (STAI) (Spielberger et al. 1970). In control subjects carefully screened for psychiatric disorders and matched for age and sex, the physiological measurements and rating scale scores were obtained just once. Analyses revealed no differences between anxiety patients and normal control subjects on hematocrit obtained under resting conditions. The two groups of anxiety patients were examined for changes following epinephrine/saline infusions. Epinephrine infusions were associated with significant increases in state anxiety, pulse, and systolic blood pressure, but not in hematocrit. No statistically significant correlations were found between hematocrit, state anxiety, pulse rate, and blood pressure under resting conditions or after epinephrine infusions.

Other experiments conducted in our laboratory involving anxiety induction with carbon dioxide inhalation and marijuana smoking (see below) did not reveal any anxiety-related changes in hematocrit. In addition, we have not found hematocrit to be a significant predictor of CBF in any of our studies (Mathew and Wilson 1987). It may be that modest hematocrit changes, within the normal physiological range, exert only minimal influence on CBF. Thus, hematocrit does not seem to be a significant factor in the determination of anxiety-related CBF changes.

Carbon Dioxide

Carbon dioxide is a potent cerebral vasodilator (Busija and Heistad 1984b; Maximilian et al. 1980; Purves 1972). Even modest changes in arterial concentrations of CO_2 are accompanied by marked alterations in CBF in a parallel direction. Changes with CMR are less consistent for both oxygen and glucose (Bryan 1990; Siesjo 1980). Anxiety is often associated with an increase in the rate of respiration and a reduction in CO_2 levels (Fried 1987;

Lader 1975). Hyperventilation and the resultant hypocapnia have been repeatedly shown to be associated with significant reductions in CBF (Gotoh et al. 1965). The decrease in CO_2 causes alkalosis, leading to reduction in oxyhemoglobin dissociation (i.e., the Bohr effect), which may reduce cerebral oxygen metabolism (Fried 1987).

Gender

We, as well as other investigators, have demonstrated higher CBF in females (Gur et al. 1982; Mathew et al. 1986). Recent studies have also reported females to have higher CMR glucose (Baxter et al. 1987a; Yoshii et al. 1988). However, it should be noted that Yoshii et al. (1988) found that when brain volume was co-varied from the CMR, male-female differences disappeared. Moreover, Hoffman et al. (1988) did not find gender differences.

Pulse Rate and Perfusion Pressure

Increase in pulse rate and elevation of blood pressure are the most common physiological changes associated with anxiety. However, these will have only limited relevance to CBF because of cerebral *autoregulation*. Autoregulation ensures a constant blood supply to the brain in spite of moderate changes in perfusion pressure (Strandgaard and Paulson 1984). However, CBF can be impaired by a profound increase or decrease in blood pressure. Also, acute changes in blood pressure can damage the blood-brain barrier, which may cause extravasation of vasoactive substances into the brain (Abdul-Rahman et al. 1979; Dahlgren et al. 1980). Lack of clarity concerning the degree to which increases in blood pressure trigger such mechanisms and the wide differences between individuals on anxiety-related blood pressure changes make the evaluation of these factors difficult.

STRESS, CEREBRAL BLOOD FLOW, AND CEREBRAL METABOLIC RATE

The concept of stress is rather diffuse and vague, and its relationship with anxiety disorders is complex. Selye (1956, p. 311) defined stress as the "non-specific response of the body to any demand made upon it," regardless of whether the demand is of a pleasant or unpleasant nature. It is also uncertain whether anxiety and the associated physiological changes can be subsumed under "non-specific response" (Lader 1982); nor is it clear to what degree studies of stress can be extrapolated to anxiety, particularly at the clinical level. However, a number of animal and human studies have been conducted in this area.

A large number of studies have been carried out with a variety of animals (but mostly with rats) to examine the effects of stress on CBF and metabolism. In these studies a variety of procedures, including restraint, ethanol withdrawal, hypotension, conditioned fear, and foot shock, have been examined. Increases in CBF and metabolism have been associated with most but not all studies. The relationships of stress to CBF and to CMR have recently been reviewed by Bryan (1990).

In animals, stress induced by immobilization for 5 to 10 minutes was found to increase CBF and cerebral metabolism by as much as twofold (Carlsson et al. 1975, 1977). However, a few investigators reported decreases in CBF in association with immobilization (Ohata et al. 1984; Rapoport et al. 1981). This reduction in CBF may have been due to hyperventilation and hypocapnia, as was pointed out earlier. The mechanism responsible for the CBF increase, on the other hand, is controversial. Epinephrine was considered responsible by some investigators, because prior adrenalectomy and/or administration of propranolol abolished this stress-induced change in CBF. Under normal conditions, epinephrine present in the peripheral blood does not cross the blood-brain barrier (Schildkraut and Kety 1967). However, the anxiety-related increase in blood pressure might disrupt the blood-brain barrier, with extravasation of epinephrine into the brain. Increase in arousal is another possible explanation.

Sharma and Dey (1986) found increased blood-brain barrier permeability after 8 hours of immobilization. However, in their study, CBF was diminished by 2% to 37% in 12 out of 14 regions. Dahlgren et al. (1981) demonstrated regional variations in the CBF response to immobilization stress. They found increased blood flow to cortical regions such as the frontal and parietal lobes and reduced flow in other brain regions such as the inferior colliculus, superior olive, hippocampus, and septal nuclei.

Lasvennes and associates (1986) compared CBF in freely moving rats and mildly restrained rats. The restrained rats showed more evidence of stress as indicated by elevated heart rate, blood pressure, and cortical flow. Frontal and parietal cortical CBF was more elevated in the freely moving rats than it was in the stressed ones. Absence of greater differences in CBF between the two groups of animals was explained on the basis of the mutually antagonistic effects of two anxiety-related factors on CBF: 1) cerebral vasoconstriction secondary to increased blood catecholamine levels, and 2) arousal-related increase in CBF.

Ledoux and co-workers (1983) measured local CBF in rats during the processing of environmental stimuli. Presentation of a tone increased CBF in the auditory pathways. However, when the animal was previously conditioned to fear the tone, blood flow additionally increased in the hypothalamus and amygdala. The increase in CBF was explained on the basis of local increases of neuronal activity.

For both normal volunteers and patients, undergoing measurements of CBF and metabolism with any technique can be stressful, and in most "normal" subjects the emotional response may not be well differentiated. When CBF is measured repeatedly, values during the second measurement tend to be lower than those in the first; no additional changes are seen after the second measurement (Warach et al. 1987). Although these CBF changes tend to be mild and often statistically nonsignificant, they do seem to represent CBF concomitants of stress reduction secondary to "getting used to" the procedure.

Gur and colleagues (1987) examined the relationship between stress (anxiety) associated with CBF and CMR measurements in two groups of normal volunteers. In the first group CBF was measured with the ^{133}Xe inhalation technique, and in the second group glucose metabolism was estimated with PET. The authors found an inverted-U relationship between CBF and anxiety measured with the STAI (Spielberger et al. 1970). Mild to moderate degrees of anxiety increased CBF, whereas more severe anxiety had the opposite effect. Gur et al. reported that CMR glucose did not have any relationship with relatively mild degrees of anxiety but that high anxiety had a negative relationship with CMR, as was seen for CBF.

Sokoloff and co-workers (1955), using the nitrous oxide inhalation technique, reported no CBF changes following administration of mental arithmetic tasks that produced peripheral sympathetic activation. Under normal conditions, changes in brain function induced with such tasks should cause an increase in CBF. The absence of such an increase suggests that sympathetic activation overshadowed this effect. Task administration was not associated with significant changes in CO_2.

In another study of the effects of mental activity, Shakhnovich and associates (1980) studied change induced by speaking and counting while measuring CBF with the hydrogen polarographic method. The test induced significant CBF increases in subjects who showed no increase in pulse rate and muscle blood flow. Increase in CBF was, however, absent in those who showed increased pulse rate and peripheral circulation. These findings support the hypothesis that a cerebral vasoconstrictor factor, probably sympathetic activation, limits the CBF increase induced by behavioral tasks.

Anticipatory anxiety and apprehension are considered normal emotions and may be defined as anticipation of the occurrence of a perceived danger. Reiman and co-workers (1989a) utilized PET measurements of regional CBF to investigate the neuroanatomic correlates of anticipatory anxiety. Measurements were obtained in eight healthy volunteers before, during, and after anticipation of a painful electric shock. Subjects were told that no shock would be delivered during the first and third measurements but that a painful electric shock would be delivered sometime within the 2-minute period after the tracer administration for the second measurement. They were also told that the severity of the shock was likely to increase with the passage of time before its arrival. During anticipation of the shock there were significant increases in subjective (i.e., STAI) and physiological measurements of anxiety. During this phase significant blood flow increases were localized in bilateral temporal poles near the anterior aspect of the lateral sulcus. Global CBF was not reported.

Rodriguez and colleagues (1989) studied the relationship between levels of anxiety and CBF measured with the ^{133}Xe inhalation technique in a group of neurologically normal patients who had no history of psychiatric illness. These patients were undergoing CBF measurements in the course of diagnostic procedures and were asked to rate their anxiety based on the STAI. Correlations were calculated between regional CBF values and ratings of anxiety. The authors reported negative correlations between level of anxiety and CBF, with the right frontal regions showing the strongest correlations.

In summary, animal studies on the effects of stress on CBF have not yielded consistent results. Although a majority of studies suggest an increase in CBF and metabolism, both decrease and increase in global CBF and regional differences have been reported. When hyperventilation and reduced CO_2 levels were controlled, the CBF change seemed to be one of increase. The precise mechanism responsible for this finding is unclear. Increase in nonspecific arousal is one possibility. The role played by disruption of the blood-brain barrier and extravasation of epinephrine is uncertain. It is unclear as to what extent these results can be extrapolated to anxiety in human subjects.

Information obtained from patients and normal subjects suggests an increase in CBF and metabolism with mild degrees of stress and anxiety. However, subjects who become severely anxious may show a decrease in CBF. This would be consistent with the concept of an arousal balance model in which there is an inverted-U–shaped relationship between stimulation and arousal level (Hebb 1955; Lindsley 1951, 1961). Based on his findings with anticipatory anxiety and the findings of others, Reiman (1990) has suggested that the poles of the temporal lobes may be the brain regions most closely associated with normal and pathological anxiety.

ANXIETY, CEREBRAL BLOOD FLOW, AND CEREBRAL METABOLIC RATE

Under Resting Conditions

The objective of studying patients with various anxiety disorders under resting conditions is to determine if in the unstimulated state there are differences in CBF or CMR among patient groups and appropriate control groups. For these studies the "resting state" is only poorly defined by descriptions of ambient laboratory conditions and by instructions to the subjects about, for example, staying awake. Some of the studies (reviewed below) utilized tasks for the subjects to perform to attempt to make laboratory conditions and subjects' activity more consistent during scans. Other studies made multiple scans, with the first being the "resting" scan, and some investigational procedure was conducted during the second or subsequent scans. For example, studies have reported resting data from the first scan of a sequence in which patients and control subjects presumably were anticipating receiving lactate infusions. No studies to date have attempted to address the possible effects these differences in methods may have played in the results, nor what role anticipatory anxiety may have had. Nonetheless, resting studies represent an important component in the total evaluation of CBF and CMR differences in anxiety disorders. Some of the studies that have been carried out in anxiety disorders to explore differences between patients and control subjects in resting CBF and CMR are summarized in Table 1–3.

We measured CBF via the ^{133}Xe inhalation technique (a two-dimensional technique) in nine right-handed subjects who met the criteria for DSM-III GAD and nine control subjects matched for age, sex, and hand preference (Mathew et al. 1982b). The participants underwent a drug washout period of 4 weeks and were required to avoid coffee, tea, and tobacco for 2 hours before the CBF measurements. The STAI was utilized to quantify levels of anxiety. CBF measurements were obtained after the subjects acclimated to the laboratory, which was kept quiet and semidark during the measurements. Because sleep has been reported to influence CBF, special care was taken to make sure that the subjects did not become drowsy during the experiment. There were no differences between anxious patients and control subjects on global and regional CBF, PE_{CO2}, pulse, and blood pressure. Pearson correlations were computed between state anxiety and CBF values in patients. Left- and right-hemispheric CBF (left hemisphere $r = -.63$, $P < .03$; right hemisphere $r = -.67$, $P < .02$) and most brain regions on both sides showed significant inverse correlations with state anxiety.

Reiman and associates (1984) studied resting CBF with PET in 10 patients with a history of panic attacks (as defined by DSM-III

[American Psychiatric Association 1980]) and 6 normal control subjects. Subsequently, all patients and 2 control subjects received an intravenous infusion of sodium lactate (10 mg per kg of 500 mM sodium DL) given over 20 to 30 minutes, and a repeat scan was performed. Resting CBF values were compared in panic disorder patients who had a panic attack following lactate infusion, patients who did not develop panic following the infusion, and normal control subjects. The three groups of subjects did not differ significantly in CBF to the whole brain, left or right hemisphere, or in the left-right ratio of hemispheric CBF. The subjects were compared with one another on left-right ratios for CBF in seven preselected regions (parahippocampal gyrus, hippocampus, hypothalamus, orbito-insular gyri, anterior cingulate gyrus, amygdala, and inferior parietal lobule). Patients who developed panic following lactate infusion showed a significantly lower right-to-left ratio in the parahippocampal gyrus as compared with the other two groups. The investigators were not able to

Table 1–3. Cerebral blood flow and metabolism: patient differences under resting conditions

Patient type[a]	Index[b]	Difference From control[c]	Reference
GAD	CBFx	ND	Mathew et al. 1982b
PD	CBFp	R ↑	Reiman et al. 1984
PD	CMR-O$_2$	GR ↑	Reiman et al. 1986
PD	CMR-GL	R ↑	Nordahl et al. 1990
OCD	CMR-GL	G ↑, R ↑	Baxter et al. 1987b
OCD	CMR-GL	G ↑, R ↑	Baxter et al. 1988
OCD	CMR-GL	G ↑, R ↑	Baxter et al. 1989
OCD	CMR-GL	R ↑	Nordahl et al. 1989
OCD[d]	CMR-GL	ND	Benkelfat et al. 1990
OCD	CMR-GL	R ↑	Swedo et al. 1989

[a]GAD = generalized anxiety disorder; PD = panic disorder; OCD = obsessive-compulsive disorder.
[b]CBFx = cerebral blood flow–xenon inhalation; CBFp = cerebral blood flow–positron-emission tomography (PET); CMR-O$_2$ = PET cerebral metabolic rate for oxygen; CMR-GL = PET cerebral metabolic rate for glucose.
[c]ND = no differences; R = regional; G = global; ↑/↓ = higher/lower than control subjects
[d]Differences from control subjects after patients were treated clinically.

determine whether this asymmetry was due to decreased left or increased right CBF values in the parahippocampal gyrus because the absolute CBF values in both regions were within the normal range. The investigators reanalyzed the data with 20 additional neurologically normal volunteers, 19 of whom showed ratios of parahippocampal blood flow identical to those of the original normal control group. One control subject, who had a high ratio comparable to that of the lactate-sensitive panic disorder patients, was found to suffer from panic disorder, and she responded to lactate infusions with panic.

Reiman and colleagues (1986) extended the findings of their first study with a larger number of subjects. In the second study, they included 16 patients with panic disorder; 8 were vulnerable to lactate-induced panic and 8 were not. Twenty-five normal control subjects were recruited for this project. The subjects included the patients and control subjects from the previous report. All subjects were physically well, and none of the subjects/patients had any other psychiatric disorders. Twelve patients were right-handed and the rest left-handed. At the time of the study, four were receiving medications, including tricyclic antidepressants and alprazolam. In addition to CBF, information concerning cerebral blood volume, cerebral oxygen extraction ratio, and metabolic rate for oxygen was obtained with PET. Once again, all measurements were made under resting conditions with subjects' eyes closed. Lactate sensitivity was verified in all patients and in 11 control subjects with a lactate infusion after the initial PET scan. PET scanning was repeated during the lactate infusion. The CBF and cerebral blood volumes were adjusted for intersubject differences in P_{ECO_2}. Again, lactate-sensitive panic disorder patients, lactate- insensitive panic disorder patients, and the control subjects were compared on CBF and CMR for oxygen indices using whole brain and regional values.

The second study replicated the original finding of asymmetry of parahippocampal blood flow in patients with panic disorder who were vulnerable to lactate infusions. However, in this study, the demarcation between the three groups of subjects on this index was not as sharp as it was in the first report. Lactate-sensitive panic disorder patients also had abnormal asymmetries of parahippocampal blood volume and metabolic rate for oxygen, with significantly lower ratios. Analysis of parahippocampal measurements on each side suggested an abnormal increase in right parahippocampal measures in the lactate-sensitive panic disorder patients. There were no significant differences between the groups in left parahippocampal indices of blood flow or metabolism; as a matter of fact, the left-hemispheric values were somewhat higher for the lactate-sensitive panic disorder group as compared with the others. Lactate-sensitive panic disorder patients also showed significantly higher whole brain metabolic rate for oxygen. This group of subjects, however, did not differ from the second group of patients on degrees of anxiety experienced during the PET scan. Correlations between anxiety levels and blood flow were not calculated.

In the first CMR glucose study of panic disorder patients, Nordahl and his associates (1990) used the PET-FDG method to examine 12 patients who met diagnostic criteria for panic disorder (DSM-III) and compared them with 30 normal control subjects. The patients were all free of any major depressive episode at the time of the scan, and all patients and subjects were free of medication. There were no differences in age, sex, or handedness between patients and control subjects. The study focused on brain regions that Reiman et al.'s work (see above) had indicated to be involved in anxiety. The patients and control subjects were studied while they performed a continuous performance auditory discrimination task; the task was performed during the uptake phase of the FDG procedure. Nordahl et al. reported hippocampal region asymmetry associated with a right-hippocampal increase in CMR for patients with panic disorder, which they felt to be consistent with Reiman et al.'s (1986) findings. They also reported for patients significant decreases in CMR in the left inferior parietal lobule and a trend toward decrease in the anterior cingulate. There was a trend toward increase in CMR in the medial orbital frontal cortex. For the patients there were no significant correlations between state anxiety (STAI; Spielberger et al. 1970) and any regional CMR values. As suggested by Nordahl et al., there is currently no method to determine what role the discrimination task played in the presentation of these differences.

The results of our study and those of Reiman and associates

are not comparable because of the substantial differences in methodology and CBF measurement techniques. We measured CBF with the ^{133}Xe inhalation technique in patients with GAD, whereas Reiman and associates utilized PET to measure CBF in lactate-sensitive and lactate-insensitive panic disorder patients. In our study, no differences were found between anxiety disorder patients and control subjects. The only positive finding was a significant inverse correlation between state anxiety and CBF. (This will be discussed in detail, together with the results of other studies involving anxiety induction, after the next subsection.)

The CBF and CMR oxygen studies done by Reiman and associates (1986) and replicated to some extent by the CMR glucose study of Nordahl et al. (1990) provide results of considerable heuristic significance. The hippocampal area has been implicated in the control of anxiety (Gray 1982). However, the physiological differences between lactate-sensitive and lactate-insensitive panic disorder are difficult to explain. The problem is further complicated by the uncertainty concerning the mechanism by which lactate induces panic. This study by Reiman et al. would need to be replicated by other laboratories with larger sample sizes before further consideration can be given to it.

Obsessive-Compulsive Disorder

Recently there have been a number of studies of CMR for glucose in patients with obsessive-compulsive disorder (OCD). Baxter and his associates have reported four studies that have examined local cerebral glucose metabolic rates in patients with OCD and compared them with those in normal control subjects and depressed patients (Baxter et al. 1985, 1987b, 1988, 1989). In one study Baxter et al. (1987b) specifically compared 14 patients who met criteria for OCD (9 of whom also met diagnostic criteria for major depression) with 14 patients with unipolar depression and 14 normal control subjects. Nine of the OCD patients were studied while medication free. The control subjects were known to the investigators and were free of physical and psychiatric illness. All were scanned using the labeled-FDG technique, and they were also rated for anxiety and depression. The OCD patients had significantly higher CMR than the depressed patients in both hemispheres globally, in the left and right caudate nuclei, and in the left orbital gyrus, with a trend toward higher levels in the right orbital gyrus. Comparisons of OCD patients with normal control subjects indicated the same pattern, but the OCD patients had a higher CMR than the control subjects in both the left and right orbital gyri. Follow-up studies of 10 OCD patients after treatment with trazodone indicated that those patients who responded to treatment ($n = 8$) failed to show significant changes in the hemispheres, caudate nuclei, or orbital gyri. However, the ratio of caudate to hemisphere metabolic rates increased in those who responded to treatment but not in the two who failed to respond. The investigators concluded that OCD patients showed regional differences of CMR compared with control subjects both before and after successful treatment.

In a second study Baxter and co-workers (1988) examined 10 OCD patients without depression and 10 normal control subjects. Again the authors reported significant differences for the hemispheres, caudate nuclei, orbital gyri, and the orbital-hemisphere ratio. These results essentially replicated findings from their previous report.

In their 1989 study Baxter et al. reported results from 14 OCD patients without depression who were compared with 10 patients with unipolar depression, 10 with bipolar depression, 10 with OCD with secondary depression, and 12 normal control subjects. The major focus of this study was to compare different groups of affective disorders; however, OCD patients without depression had higher CMR than both normal subjects and OCD patients with depression. OCD patients with depression tended to have higher CMR than did control subjects, while the two depressed groups had lower CMR than did normal subjects (Baxter et al. 1989).

In what the authors described as a replication with improvements of Baxter et al.'s findings, Nordahl et al. (1989) studied 8 nondepressed OCD patients and 30 normal control subjects, using the PET-FDG method. One major difference in methods is that Nordahl et al. employed an auditory continuous performance task during the scan that required sustained attention. Nordahl et al. did not find differences in normalized global metabolic rates of the basal ganglia structures between these two groups of subjects; however, they did find higher regional CMR in both the left and right orbital frontal cortex in OCD patients, which is consistent with the previous findings of Baxter et al. (1989).

In a follow-up study Nordahl and colleagues (Benkelfat et al. 1990) repeated the scans of 8 OCD patients who were treated with clomipramine for at least 12 weeks (mean = 16.1 weeks). While there were no differences in global gray matter CMR between an off-drug period and during treatment, there were significant decreases in left caudate and orbital frontal areas. There was also a trend for greater change in the left caudate for those patients who responded to treatment. When the posttreatment scans were compared with the scans for the 30 control subjects from Nordahl et al.'s (1989) previous study, none of the previously reported differences were still significant. The authors concluded that there was an association between clinical improvement and a return to a "more normal" level of CMR in the orbital frontal cortex and caudate. This trend toward normalization of CMR after successful treatment is consistent with that reported by Baxter et al. (1987b).

In a PET study of childhood onset of OCD, Swedo et al. (1989) compared CMR glucose in 18 OCD patients with 18 age- and sex-matched control subjects. The authors reported a significant positive correlation between severity of illness and changes in CMR in the right orbital area. They also reported differences between OCD patients and control subjects in a number of areas of both the left and right prefrontal cortex, as well as evidence of differences in the cingulate gyrus. Consistent with other reports, they found some increases in CMR with clinical improvement following treatment.

It is difficult to compare the results of studies of OCD among themselves or directly with those of other diagnostic groups because of differences in methods and control groups. For example, Baxter et al. reported absolute values, whereas Nordahl et al. reported normalized values, and there is no way to determine the effect of the performance task compared with the resting scans. Nonetheless, there appears to be agreement in the pattern of findings, with OCD patients having higher metabolic values in some regions as compared with control subjects. Baxter (1990) has proposed, based on available data, that the orbital cortex and striatum are dysfunctional in OCD. Nordahl et al. (1990) point out that there are similarities between the results for panic disorder and OCD patients. These similarities include CMR decreases in the inferior parietal region and at least a trend toward increases in the orbital frontal region.

Cerebral Blood Flow and Cerebral Metabolic Rate Changes Associated With Anxiety Induction

Cerebral blood flow is influenced by a variety of factors and, therefore, shows a significant degree of variation among subjects (Mathew et al. 1986). On the other hand, CBF within the same individual tends to be more stable over time (Blauenstein et al. 1977), and, thus, measurements made before and after anxiety induction would seem to be a useful approach. The effects on CBF of a variety of agents and techniques known to increase anxiety have been examined. Some of the studies that have employed anxiety induction to evaluate differences between patients and control subjects are summarized in Table 1–4.

Caffeine is one of the most widely used psychotropic agents, and it is known to induce anxiety in normal subjects and in patients with anxiety disorders (Charney et al. 1985; Veleber and Templer 1984). We examined the effect of orally administered caffeine on CBF and anxiety (Mathew and Wilson 1985). Twenty-four physically and mentally healthy normal volunteers who were medication free for a period of 2 weeks prior to the study participated. The subjects abstained from all caffeine-containing substances for a minimum of 2 hours before the experiment. CBF measurements were obtained with the ^{133}Xe inhalation technique three times in each subject under identical laboratory conditions. Immediately after the first measurement, the subjects received either 250 mg of caffeine, or a placebo, with lemonade under double-blind conditions. The drug/placebo administrations were completed in less than 5 minutes. Subjects were assigned to the caffeine and placebo groups on a random basis; 14 subjects received caffeine and 10, placebo. CBF measurements were repeated twice more: 30 minutes and 90 minutes after the administration of the caffeine/placebo. During the CBF measurements,

Table 1–4. Cerebral blood flow changes associated with anxiety induction

Subjects[a]	Index[b]	Stimulant	Index change[c]	Related to anxiety[d]	References
N	CBFx	Caffeine	G↓	No	Mathew and Wilson 1985
N	CBFx	Scan procedure	G↓↑	Yes	Gur et al. 1987[e]
GAD, PD, N	CBFx	Caffeine	G↓	No	Mathew and Wilson 1990
PD, N	CBFp	Caffeine	G↓	No	Cameron et al. 1990
GAD	CBFx	Epinephrine	ND	Yes	Mathew and Wilson 1989b
GAD, N	CBFx	CO_2 (5%)	G↑	Yes	Mathew and Wilson 1988
PD	CBFx	Acetazolamide	G↑	Yes	Mathew et al. 1989b
ND	CBFx	Marijuana	G↓	Yes	Mathew et al. 1989a
PD, N	CBFs	Sodium lactate	G↑	Yes	Stewart et al. 1988
PD	CBFp	Sodium lactate	R↑	Yes	Reiman et al. 1984
PD	CBFp	Sodium lactate	R↑	Yes	Reiman et al. 1986
PD	CBFs	Behavioral	ND	No	Woods et al. 1988
OCD	CBFx	Behavioral Imaginal flooding In vivo exposure	R↑ R↓,G↑	Yes	Zohar et al. 1989
Phobia	CBFp	Behavioral	ND	No	Mountz et al. 1989

[a]N = normal; GAD = generalized anxiety disorder; PD = panic disorder; OCD = obsessive-compulsive disorder.
[b]CBFx = cerebral blood flow–xenon inhalation; CBFp = cerebral blood flow–positron-emission tomography (PET); CBFs = cerebral blood flow–single-photon emission computed tomography (SPECT).
[c]ND = no difference; R = regional; G = global; ↑/↓ = increase/decrease.
[d]Indicates whether changes in anxiety were reported to be in the direction of or correlated with cerebral blood flow.
[e]This study also looked at cerebral metabolic rate—glucose and found a decrease with anxiety.

blood pressure, respiratory rate, PE_{CO_2}, and a one-channel electroencephalographic recording were monitored. After each CBF measurement, levels of anxiety were quantified with the State Anxiety Scale of the STAI.

Analyses indicated a statistically significant decrease in CBF following caffeine after both 30 minutes and 90 minutes. There was, however, no significant decrease in CBF following saline. These findings were substantiated by post hoc testing that indicated no differences between the two groups on resting CBF and among the three sets of CBF in the placebo group. PE_{CO_2}, blood pressure, respiratory rate, and state anxiety did not differentiate among the three groups and were stable across the three measurements in both groups.

In another study (Mathew and Wilson 1990), CBF was measured before and 15 minutes after 250 mg of caffeine was given intravenously to eight drug-free patients (for 2 weeks prior to start of study) with GAD and to nine patients with panic disorder (as defined by DSM-III-R [American Psychiatric Association 1987]) as well as to nine normal volunteers. Another nine volunteers received double-blind intravenous injections of saline. The subjects were also questioned about the DSM-III-R symptoms of panic immediately after the experiment and 24 hours later by telephone. The four groups of subjects who participated in the study did not differ significantly on age or sex distribution. Caffeine administration was associated with statistically significant decreases in CBF (−22.3% of the baseline), but there were no changes after placebo. Caffeine did not bring about significant changes in PE_{CO_2}. The decrease in CBF was similar in all brain regions for the three caffeine groups. Caffeine did not cause any significant changes in the state anxiety (as measured by the STAI) in patients; however, the normal control subjects who received caffeine reported an increase in anxiety. None of the participants reported panic attacks after the drug or placebo for up to 24 hours. It is possible that the dose of caffeine used was too low to induce significant increases in anxiety.

Cameron et al. (1990) studied CBF with PET in four patients with panic disorder and four normal control subjects following intravenous administration of caffeine (dose range = 120–350 mg). Consistent with the above findings, there was a significant global decrease in CBF but no regional differences. There was no significant change in rated anxiety for patients or control subjects.

Cerebral vasoconstriction induced by caffeine (Mathew and Wilson 1985) is in keeping with previous reports (Mathew et al. 1983). However, this change in CBF was independent of changes in state anxiety and indices of sympathetic activity. In fact, in spite of the significant reduction in CBF following caffeine, there were no changes in state anxiety, blood pressure, pulse rate, or respiratory rate. However, it should be noted that other investigators have reported significant elevation in anxiety following the administration of caffeine at comparable and even lower doses (Veleber and Templer 1984). The most important finding of the study is that caffeine, which can induce anxiety, also induces cerebral vasoconstriction. However, the study does not warrant any conclusions about the relationship between cerebral vasoconstrictive and anxiogenic properties of caffeine. Perhaps caffeine given at much higher doses might have induced both anxiety and cerebral vasoconstriction.

Epinephrine is known to induce anxiety in predisposed people (Gorman 1987). We measured CBF before and 2 minutes after intravenous infusions of epinephrine or saline given under double-blind conditions in 40 patients with GAD (Mathew and Wilson 1989b). Twenty patients received epinephrine (0.2 µg/kg) and 20 others received saline. The subjects were assigned to the two groups on a random basis, and the infusions were given under double-blind conditions. CBF measurements were obtained using the ^{133}Xe inhalation technique with the other routine quantifications and precautions. Anxiety experienced during the CBF measurements was measured with the State Anxiety Scale of the STAI.

Epinephrine infusions were followed by significant increases in state anxiety, respiration, and pulse rate, and by nonsignificant decreases in P_{ECO_2}. Saline infusions, on the other hand, were not associated with any changes. There were no significant differences between the epinephrine and saline groups on hemispheric or regional CBF before and after the infusions. Correction for differences in P_{ECO_2} did not alter the results (Maximilian et al. 1980). The relationships between changes in state anxiety, the physiological indices, and CBF were examined with Pearson correlations in both groups. In the epinephrine group, inverse correlations were found between state anxiety and CBF (right hemisphere, $r = -.51$, $P < .05$; left hemisphere, $r = -.52$, $P < .05$), whereas in the saline group the relationship was positive (right hemisphere, $r = .50$, $P < .05$; left hemisphere, $r = .44$, $P < .05$). $PEco_2$ correlated significantly with global CBF in the saline group ($r = .42$, $P < .05$) but not in the epinephrine group ($r = .14$).

The findings in the saline group are more straightforward and easy to explain. As was pointed out earlier, $PEco_2$ changes are widely known to be associated with parallel CBF changes (Maximilian et al. 1980). Similarly, anxiety-related increase in arousal can account for the CBF increase. The situation, however, is much more complicated in the epinephrine group. In that group, which showed significant increases in state anxiety, there was an inverse correlation between anxiety and CBF. The normally close association between CBF and $PEco_2$ was distorted. The results of this study would seem to suggest that mild increases in state anxiety tend to increase CBF (placebo group), while marked elevation in anxiety is associated with CBF decrease (epinephrine group). The factor or factors responsible for such a CBF decrease might also account for the distorted relationship between CO_2 and CBF (Mathew and Wilson 1988). As was pointed out earlier, sympathetic activation may be this anxiety-related vasoconstrictive factor.

Carbon dioxide inhalation is another technique utilized by several investigators to induce anxiety in patients with anxiety disorders (Gorman et al. 1984; van den Hout and Griez 1984; Woods et al. 1986). We examined CBF and mood changes induced by inhalation of 5% CO_2 in nine patients with GAD and in a sex-matched group of normal control subjects of comparable age (Mathew and Wilson 1988). All subjects were right-handed and in good physical health. They were medication-free for a minimum of 2 weeks prior to start of the study and avoided coffee and tobacco for 3 hours before the experiment. CBF was measured twice at an interval of 30 minutes with the standard measurement technique and usual precautions in all subjects. All subjects inhaled a mixture of 5% CO_2 in room air for 2 minutes before and during the second CBF measurement. Anxiety experienced by the subjects during the CBF measurements was quantified with the STAI, and a short rating scale was utilized to measure somatic symptoms of anxiety (Tyrer 1976).

There were no group differences in blood pressure, pulse, respiratory rate, hematocrit, and PE_{CO_2}. However, as would be expected, significant increases in PE_{CO_2}, equivalent for both groups, were found. Although anxious patients had significantly higher state anxiety during both measurements, no significant difference between the two groups on change in state anxiety emerged. Both groups reported difficulty in breathing. Although initial analyses indicated no CBF differences between the groups, inspection of the data indicated that approximately half the subjects (patients and control subjects) had a decrease in anxiety scores (−8.0 units of STAI, SD = 4.9), while the remaining subjects had an increase in anxiety (+7.2 units, SD = 4.9) following CO_2 administration. The latter group also showed a significant increase in somatic symptoms of anxiety during the second run ($t = 2.1$, $P < .05$). There were no differences between the two groups on PE_{CO_2} during the second measurement. Further examination showed that there was a consistent pattern of CBF change. For both patients and control subjects, those who had a decrease in anxiety scores had a statistically significantly greater increase of CBF than did those who had an increase in state anxiety.

Lack of an anxiety response to CO_2 inhalation was surprising. Although CO_2 inhalation has been reported to increase anxiety (van den Hout and Griez 1984), it has also been reported to relieve anxiety (Ley and Walker 1973). Subjects who reported anxiety also reported significantly more somatic symptoms, especially difficulty in breathing, confirming the previous observation that peripheral symptoms induced by CO_2 trigger central feelings of anxiety in predisposed people (Griez and van den Hout 1982). CO_2 increased CBF in both anxious patients and control subjects in an identical manner. However, when patients and control subjects who became anxious were separated from those who did not, significant differences emerged. Those who reported anxiety showed less marked CBF increase as compared with those who did not.

Acetazolamide is known to inhibit carbonic anhydrase (which

normally catalyses the hydration of CO_2 and the hydrolysis of carbonic acid) and to induce hypercarbia. We studied anxiety (as measured by the STAI), physiological changes, and CBF before and after double-blind intravenous injection of either 1 g of acetazolamide ($n = 13$) or saline ($n = 10$) in drug-free (for 4 weeks prior to start of study) panic disorder patients (Mathew et al. 1989b). The patients were questioned about DSM-III-R symptoms of panic immediately after the experiment and 24 hours later. None of the participants reported panic attacks following drug administration, and there was no significant change in somatic symptoms or state anxiety after acetazolamide. Subjects who received acetazolamide showed highly significant increases in CBF. When patients who reported increased anxiety were separated from those who did not, the former showed less marked cerebral vasodilation—a result that is similar to the findings of the CO_2 inhalation study.

Once again, there appears to be a cerebral vasoconstrictive factor related to anxiety that seems to distort the relationship between CBF and CO_2 in subjects who become anxious. Busija and Heistad (1984a) showed that electric and reflex activation of the sympathetic nervous system reduces CBF and increases cerebral vascular resistance during hypercarbia in anesthetized cats and awake dogs. The same mechanism might be responsible for the limited CBF response to CO_2 in anxious subjects (Mathew and Wilson 1989a).

Marijuana has sympathomimetic properties and often induces anxiety and panic in inexperienced users (Benedikt et al. 1986; Nahas et al. 1984; Weil 1970). We measured CBF before and after marijuana smoking in experienced (i.e., a minimum of 10 "joints" a week for 3 years) and inexperienced subjects (i.e., no marijuana for a minimum of 3 years) (Mathew et al. 1989a). The subjects were physically and mentally healthy and medication free for a minimum of 1 month prior to study. They avoided alcohol and marijuana for 12 hours (experienced smokers) and coffee and tobacco for 3 hours before the experiments.

CBF measurements were made with the ^{133}Xe inhalation technique using the standard procedure with the usual precautions. Anxiety experienced during CBF measurements was quantified with the STAI. A high-potency marijuana cigarette (THC 2.2%)

was administered 60 minutes before the second CBF measurement. CBF was measured twice at an interval of 60 minutes in 15 inexperienced smokers under resting conditions. The remaining 26 subjects (9 experienced and 17 inexperienced smokers) smoked a high-potency marijuana cigarette (THC 2.2%) 60 minutes before the second CBF measurement. Mood changes during CBF measurements were quantified with the Profile of Mood States (McNair et al. 1971). Measurements of CBF before and after marijuana inhalation in experienced and inexperienced smokers were compared (using multivariate analysis of variance) with measurements of control subjects, who had two resting CBF runs. Inexperienced smokers showed significant CBF decreases in all regions after marijuana inhalation; there were no significant regional differences. The experienced smokers, on the other hand, showed a CBF increase in both hemispheres. Inexperienced smokers had significant increases in blood pressure, pulse rate, respiration, and state anxiety, and the experienced smokers had significant increases in diastolic blood pressure and pulse rate.

The results of this study indicate an increase in state anxiety following marijuana smoking in inexperienced smokers. This finding is further validated by the significant postmarijuana increases in pulse rate, blood pressure, and respiration in this group. For the combined inexperienced and experienced groups, state anxiety showed significant inverse correlations with CBF. The results of this study are in keeping with the other CBF/anxiety-induction studies described above: all indicated the existence of an anxiety-related cerebral vasoconstrictive factor.

Stewart and co-workers (1988) measured CBF with SPECT in 10 drug-free patients with panic disorder and 5 normal control subjects. Measurements were obtained when the patients were at rest or during saline or sodium lactate infusions. Lactate induced panic in 6 patients and none of the control subjects. All participants showed an increase in CBF during lactate infusions. However, patients who panicked showed less of an increase or even a decrease in CBF. Changes in CBF and severity of panic did not correlate. The effect of hypocapnia on the CBF reduction could not be assessed because the investigators did not measure CO_2.

Woods and colleagues (1988) measured regional CBF with SPECT after intravenous injections of 0.4 mg/kg of yohimbine and saline, on separate days, in six drug-free patients with panic disorder and six control subjects. Yohimbine decreased bilateral frontal cortical blood flow (relative to the rest of the brain) consistently in comparison with placebo in the patients but not in the control subjects. Panic disorder patients experienced higher anxiety levels after administration of yohimbine.

The results of other studies involving lactate infusion—those by Reiman and associates (1984, 1986)—have been presented above (see subsection on CBF studies of anxiety under resting conditions). Reiman et al. (1989b) have more recently measured regional CBF with PET in patients with panic disorder (DSM-III-R) and normal control subjects before and during lactate infusion. During the infusion, 8 patients had anxiety attacks, whereas 9 patients and 15 control subjects did not. With the exception of 1 patient, the participants were medication free for 2 weeks prior to the study. Patients who panicked had a significantly greater increase in the number of anxiety symptoms and in systolic and diastolic blood pressure, and a significantly greater decrease in arterial CO_2 levels during lactate infusion. They also showed significant increases in CBF bilaterally in the temporofrontal cortex, bilaterally in the insular cortex, in the claustrum, bilaterally in or near the superior colliculus, and in or near the left anterior cerebellar vermis. Lactate infusion was not associated with significant changes in regional CBF in the nonpanicking patients or control subjects. Global CBF was not reported.

Zohar and associates (1989) evaluated CBF changes associated with anxiety in patients with OCD. CBF was measured with the ^{133}Xe inhalation technique under three conditions: relaxation, imaginal flooding, and in vivo exposure to a phobic stimulus. During the relaxation run, subjects listened to a taped description of a relaxation scene. Imaginal flooding consisted of auditory presentation of a verbal description tailored to the patient's "contamination fear." In vivo exposure consisted of applying a specific contamination object to the dorsum of the right hand of each patient while he or she listened to the tape that was used during imaginal flooding. Subjective ratings of anxiety showed incremental increase from the relaxation, to imaginal flooding, to in vivo exposure. Parallel changes were also seen in blood pressure (systolic and diastolic) and heart rate; however, P_{ECO_2} did not show significant changes during the three runs. Global CBF showed a nonsignificant increase during imaginal flooding, with the increase in CBF in the temporal cortex (both sides together) reaching significance. However, in vivo exposure was associated with significant decrease in global and all regional flow values.

Mountz and co-workers (1989) also utilized PET to examine the effect of state anxiety on CBF. Seven right-handed, premenopausal females with a history of animal phobia (DSM-III) and a control population of eight age-matched females participated in the project. All subjects were drug free for a period of 1 month prior to the study. CBF measurements were performed five times: 1) at rest, 2) during confrontation with the phobic object, 3) at rest again, 4) a second time during confrontation, and, once again, 5) at rest. The phobic stimuli produced marked and repeated increases in both the objective and subjective measures of anxiety. There were no significant differences in these measures between the three rest scans or the two confrontation scans. The physiological variables that showed significant changes included increases in heart rate and blood pressure and a decrease in arterial levels of CO_2. Analysis of absolute global and regional CBF showed significant differences across rest and confrontation scans, with lower values being found in the two confrontation scans. There were no significant blood flow differences among the rest scans or the confrontation scans. The data were reanalyzed after correcting the CBF for the hypocapnia using an experimentally established equation. This analysis failed to show global or regional blood flow differences between the confrontation and rest scans.

The number of studies on CBF changes associated with anxiety induction is too small to draw firm conclusions. However, it seems safe to state that all available studies indicate a cerebral vasoconstrictive factor associated with severe anxiety. Anxiety induced by epinephrine infusions in patients with GAD correlated inversely with global CBF. Patients who became anxious after CO_2 inhalation and panic disorder patients after administration of acetazolamide showed less CBF increase compared with those who did not become anxious. Anxiety induced by marijuana smoking in inexperienced users was associated with a decrease in CBF. Panic disorder patients who panicked after lactate infusions had less increase or even a decrease in CBF. Induction of anxiety with yohimbine in panic disorder patients was associated with a decrease in frontal flow bilaterally. Severe anxiety induced by in vivo exposure to a feared object decreased CBF in patients with OCD. Although hypocapnia could account for the CBF decrease in some studies, in several others it could not.

Buchsbaum and associates (1987) conducted a PET study on the effects of benzodiazepines on CMR glucose in patients with anxiety disorders. Eighteen patients with GAD (DSM-III) entered a 21-day, double-blind, placebo-controlled random assignment trial of clorazepate. CMR was measured before and after the treatment. Posttreatment values indicated a decrease in CMR in the visual cortex and a relative increase in CMR in the basal ganglia and thalamus. A correlation between regional CMR changes and regional benzodiazepine receptor binding density (from other human autopsy studies) was observed.

Studies on stress and CBF conducted by two groups of investigators also suggest similar conclusions. Sokoloff and co-workers (1955) reported no CBF changes following mental arithmetic task administration that induced peripheral sympathetic activation. The nitrous oxide inhalation technique for CBF measurement was utilized. Under normal conditions, changes in brain function associated with the tasks should cause an increase in CBF. Its absence suggests that sympathetic activation overshadowed this cerebral vasodilation. Shakhnovich and colleagues (1980) studied CBF changes induced by mental activity (i.e., speaking and counting) using the hydrogen polarographic method. The test induced diffuse CBF increases in subjects who showed no increase in pulse rate and muscle blood flow. The increase in CBF was, however, absent in those subjects who showed increased pulse rate and peripheral circulation. These findings support our hypothesis that a cerebral vasoconstrictive factor, probably sympathetic activation, limits the CBF increase induced by behavioral tasks.

Reivich and co-workers (1983) examined the association between anxiety and CMR for glucose in 18 right-handed males. Anxiety levels were measured with the STAI. The authors found a curvilinear relationship between anxiety and frontocortical metabolic rates. A quadratic function fit the data for the state anxiety significantly better than a linear function. Frontal metabolism seemed to increase as a function of anxiety up to a point, after which greater anxiety was associated with decreased metabolic activity. This pattern was not seen in other brain regions. When the subjects were divided into high-anxious and low-anxious groups, an interaction between anxiety and the metabolic rates in the two hemispheres was found.

SUMMARY

Nonspecific arousal mediated by the reticular formation is believed to be an important component of anxiety. Conditions associated with increase and decrease in arousal are associated with parallel changes in global CBF. Stimulation and destruction of the brain-stem region that houses the reticular formation are associated with increase and decrease in CBF, respectively. The frontal lobe is the cortical apparatus responsible for the maintenance of arousal. Under resting conditions, frontal regions show higher perfusion than do other cortical regions. However, the concept of hyperfrontality of CBF distribution under resting conditions is controversial because this phenomenon has not been replicated by most studies using three-dimensional techniques.

The relationship between CBF, CMR, and anxiety is complicated by the multiple factors that influence the former two and the widespread physiological changes that accompany the latter. Anxiety-related factors (other than arousal) such as plasma catecholamines, sympathetic nervous system, blood viscosity, and CO_2 levels can influence CBF and CMR.

Investigators have reported increases in CBF following the administration of epinephrine. This effect does not appear to be due to the vasoactive properties of the drug, but the precise mechanism is unclear. Cerebral blood vessels receive sympathetic innervation from the superior cervical ganglion. Stimulation of these fibers causes cerebral vasoconstriction. Thus, the anxiety-related increase in sympathetic activity might result in reduced cerebral perfusion. CBF and blood viscosity are inversely related. However, studies conducted in our laboratory have thus far failed to confirm previous reports of stress polycytosis, and, furthermore, mild changes in hematocrit do not appear to affect CBF.

Normal subjects and anxious patients do not show significant differences on global CBF under resting conditions. However, patients with panic disorder who are prone to develop panic attacks during lactate infusion exhibit asymmetry of blood flow to the parahippocampal regions. These results are also shown in patients with OCD, in whom there is evidence that the orbital frontal cortex and striatum may be dysfunctional. Differences in regional CMR from that of control subjects appear to be present in OCD in both the symptomatic and treated states.

The effect of acute anxiety on CBF is complex. Mild anxiety (and arousal) seems to increase CBF and CMR. Several lines of evidence support reduction of CBF and CMR with severe anxiety. Resting CBF and anxiety levels correlated inversely in patients with GAD. CBF and anxiety levels also showed negative correlations when anxiety was induced by intravenous infusion of epinephrine in anxiety disorder patients. CO_2 is a potent cerebral vasodilator, and acute anxiety is often associated with rapid breathing and hypocapnia. Increase in CBF induced by CO_2 and acetazolamide injections was less marked in patients and control subjects who reported increased anxiety. Subjects who showed severe anxiety following marijuana inhalation exhibited CBF reductions.

Patients who panicked following lactate infusion showed either less increase or a decrease in CBF. Anxiety precipitated by intravenous injections of yohimbine in panic patients was associated with reduced frontal flow. Patients with OCD showed a decrease in CBF during anxiety that was induced by exposure to a feared object. Furthermore, subjects who experienced severe anxiety during measurements of CBF and CMR glucose (using PET) showed inverse correlations between their anxiety and CBF/CMR.

The mechanism responsible for this CBF and CMR reduction during severe anxiety is unclear. Hypocapnia would seem to be the most likely explanation; however, several studies in which CO_2 was measured could not explain the CBF reduction on this basis. Anxiety-related increase in sympathetic cerebral vasoconstrictive tone is another factor to be considered, but it cannot explain the CMR changes. Conclusions in this regard would be premature.

The inverted-U relationship between anxiety and CBF/CMR (i.e., increase in CBF with mild anxiety and decrease in CBF with severe anxiety) is of considerable heuristic significance. CBF and CMR are both indices of brain function, and, thus, this finding seems to support previous reports of an inverted-U relationship between performance and anxiety levels.

Reiman and associates (1989a, 1989b) argue that both anticipatory anxiety and lactate-induced panic attacks involve the same regions of the temporal pole bilaterally. They have provided data on specific brain regions that might be involved in the mediation of anxiety and panic. Their findings have been in part replicated in the studies of OCD by other groups. Although of great interest, these findings need further replication and confirmation.

Anxious patients frequently report symptoms suggestive of cerebral ischemia. Preservation of cerebral metabolism is vital to life, and a number of mechanisms protect the brain from becoming ischemic even in the face of decreased CBF. CBF has to be reduced by approximately 50% of normal (below 20 ml/100 g/minute) for ischemia to result (Adler et al. 1971; Lassen and Astrup 1987). The degree of CBF reduction found to accompany induced anxiety is not substantial enough to produce cerebral ischemia (Frackowiak 1985). However, it is possible that certain anxiety disorder patients may develop cerebral vasospasm and cerebral ischemia. Oversensitivity to sympathetic stimulation has been implicated in cerebral vasospasm (Boullin 1980; Rosenblum and Guilianti 1973), and anxious patients have been shown to have heightened sensitivity to sympathetic activation (Nesse et al. 1984).

Cerebral blood flow during acute anxiety will depend upon the interplay of central (i.e., arousal) and peripheral (i.e., sympathetic tone, CO_2, etc.) factors. The extensive volume of literature on the psychophysiology of anxiety indicates wide variations between and within subjects. In all probability, this will also be true of cerebral circulation. The CBF changes associated with anxiety are likely to depend upon a number of factors, some of which are discussed here. There are other factors about which very little is known (e.g., effects of neurotransmitters, intracerebral blood vessel innervation).

FUTURE DIRECTIONS

Future studies should take into account the multiple mechanisms by which anxiety may influence CBF and CMR. This would include arousal, autonomic nervous system, CO_2, and blood viscosity. CO_2 would seem to be the most serious source of confusion because of its profound effect on blood flow, the marked changes during acute anxiety, the nonlinear relationship between CO_2 and CBF, and intersubject (different age groups) and regional (gray matter vs. white matter) variability on the relationship between CO_2 and CBF. Regional CBF and CMR changes might vary between psychic and somatic subtypes of anxiety since the central and peripheral changes influence CBF differently (Morrow and Labrum 1978; Tyrer 1976). Furthermore, perceptions of the bodily symptoms of anxiety should increase CBF and CMR in brain regions that mediate that function. In view of the intersubject variability in the physiology of anxiety and the multiple mechanisms by which anxiety can influence CBF, small-scale studies are unlikely to yield meaningful information. Many of the studies reviewed above involved induction of anxiety with a variety of pharmacological agents. It is conceivable that some of those agents may have had direct effects (independent of their anxiogenic or anxiolytic action) on CBF. Use of behavioral techniques to induce and relieve anxiety may yield different data.

It is well recognized that specific cortical areas show increased activity when a subject is engaged in a task. The task can be as simple as having the subject look at a checkerboard display, or more complex, such as requiring the subject to make decisions. For example, investigators are now using continuous-performance tasks (particular in PET-FDG scans), with the objective of making the scanning environment more constant. There is much to be said that is positive about the use of tasks to standardize the testing procedures. However, no accounting of the effects of these tasks has been taken in such issues as computations of regional changes when these changes are expressed as a ratio of whole brain or hemispheric values, even though there may be clear regional and hemispheric effects. Nor has there been an accounting of the possible differences that various patient groups may show as a function of their illness in response to these tasks.

Nor has it been shown how the tasks may impact the results. In anxiety disorders some accounting of the effects of stress induced by these procedures needs to be made, and study designs must reflect the potential impact. For example, where possible, one may need to arrange the experimental conditions for repeated testing so that the effects (e.g., baseline effects) are distributed across the repeated measures (e.g., by using crossover or latin-square designs).

Finally, it is important to explore such factors as present clinical state (e.g., rated level of anxiety), duration of illness, and response to treatment as they relate to changes in regional CBF and CMR. For example, it is important to determine if there appear to be permanent alterations of brain structure in anxiety disorders such as those seen in other disorders (e.g., MRI studies in schizophrenia). It is also important to assess whether there is evidence for progressive change as a function of duration of illness or whether the alterations are state dependent and possibly responsive to treatment.

REFERENCES

Abdul-Rahman A, Dahlgren N, Johansson BB, et al: Increase in local cerebral blood flow induced by circulating adrenalin: involvement of blood-brain barrier dysfunction. Acta Physiol Scand 107:227–232, 1979

Ackner B: The relationship between anxiety and the level of peripheral vasomotor activity. J Psychosom Res 1:21–48, 1956

Adler R, MacRitchie K, Engel GL: Psychological processes and ischemic stroke. Psychosom Med 33:1–29, 1971

American Psychiatric Association: Diagnostic and Statistical Manual of Mental Disorders, 3rd Edition. Washington, DC, American Psychiatric Association, 1980

American Psychiatric Association: Diagnostic and Statistical Manual of Mental Disorders, 3rd Edition, Revised. Washington, DC, American Psychiatric Association, 1987

Ax AF: The physiological differentiation between fear and anger. Psychosom Med 15:433–442, 1953

Barlett EJ, Brodie JD, Wolf AP, et al: Reproducibility of cerebral metabolic measurements in resting human subjects. J Cereb Blood Flow Metab 8:502–512, 1988

Baxter LR: Brain imaging as a tool in establishing a theory of brain pathology in obsessive-compulsive disorder. J Clin Psychiatry 51(no 2, suppl):22–25, 1990

Baxter LR, Phelps ME, Mazziotta JC, et al: Cerebral metabolic rate for glucose in mood disorders studied with PET and (F-18)-fluorodeoxyglucose (FDG). Arch Gen Psychiatry 42:441–447, 1985

Baxter LR, Mazziotta JC, Phelps ME, et al: Cerebral glucose metabolic rates in normal human females and males. Psychiatry Res 21:237–245, 1987a

Baxter LR, Phelps ME, Mazziotta JC, et al: Local cerebral glucose metabolic rates in obsessive-compulsive disorder. Arch Gen Psychiatry 44:211–218, 1987b

Baxter LR, Schwartz JM, Mazziotta JC, et al: Cerebral glucose metabolic rates in non-depressed patients with obsessive-compulsive disorder. Am J Psychiatry 145:1560–1563, 1988

Baxter LR, Schwartz JM, Phelps ME, et al: Reduction of prefrontal cortex glucose metabolism common to three types of depression. Arch Gen Psychiatry 46:243–250, 1989

Benedikt RA, Cristofaro P, Mendelson JH: Effects of acute marijuana smoking in post-menopausal women. Psychopharmacology (Berlin) 90:14–17, 1986

Benitone J, Kling A: Polycythemia of stress in psychiatric hospital populations. J Psychosom Res 14:105–108, 1970

Benkelfat C, Nordahl TE, Semple WE, et al: Local cerebral glucose metabolic rates in obsessive-compulsive disorder. Arch Gen Psychiatry 47:840–848, 1990

Blauenstein UW, Halsey JH, Wilson EM, et al: [133]Xenon inhalation method, analysis of reproducibility: some of its physiological implications. Stroke 8:92–102, 1977

Boullin DJ: Cerebral Vasospasm. New York, Wiley, 1980

Broderson P, Paulson OB, Bolgic TC, et al: Cerebral hyperemia during epileptic seizures in man. Arch Neurol 28:334–338, 1973

Bryan RM: Cerebral blood flow and energy metabolism during stress. Am J Physiol 259:H269–H280, 1990

Buchsbaum MS, Ingvar DH, Kessler R, et al: Cerebral glucography with positron tomography: use in normal subjects and inpatients with schizophrenia. Arch Gen Psychiatry 39:251–259, 1982

Buchsbaum MS, Wu J, Haier R, et al: Positron emission tomography assessment of effects of benzodiazepines on regional glucose metabolic rate in patients with anxiety disorder. Life Sci 40:2393–2400, 1987

Busija DW, Heistad DD: Effects of activation of the sympathetic nerves on cerebral blood flow during hypercarbia in cats and rabbits. J Physiol 347:35–45, 1984a

Busija DW, Heistad DD: Factors involved in the physiological regulation of the cerebral circulation. Rev Physiol Biochem Pharmacol 101:161–211, 1984b

Cameron OG, Modell JG, Hariharan M: Caffeine and human cerebral blood flow: a positron emission tomography study. Life Sci 47:1141–1146, 1990

Carlsson C, Hagerdal M, Siesjo BK: Increase in cerebral oxygen uptake and blood flow in immobilization stress. Acta Physiol Scand 95:206–208, 1975

Carlsson C, Hagerdal M, Kaasik AE, et al: A catecholamine mediated increase in cerebral oxygen uptake during immobilization stress in rat. Brain Res 119:223–231, 1977

Carpenter MB: Human Neuroanatomy, 7th Edition. Baltimore, MD, Williams & Wilkins, 1976, pp 547–599

Charney DS, Heninger GR, Jatlow PI: Increased anxiogenic effects of caffeine in panic disorders. Arch Gen Psychiatry 42:233–243, 1985

Dahlgren N, Rosen I, Sakabe T, et al: Cerebral functional, metabolic and circulatory effects of intravenous infusion of adrenalin in the rat. Brain Res 184:143–152, 1980

Dahlgren N, Ingvar M, Yokoyama H, et al: Influence of nitrous oxide on local cerebral blood flow in awake, minimally restrained rats. J Cereb Blood Flow Metab 1:143–152, 1981

Dameshek W: Stress erythrocytosis. Blood 8:282–289, 1953

Deutsch G, Eisenberg HM: Frontal blood flow changes in recovery from coma. J Cereb Blood Flow Metab 7:29–34, 1987

Devous MD, Stokely EM, Chehabi HH, et al: Normal distribution of regional cerebral blood flow measured by dynamic single-photon emission tomography. J Cereb Blood Flow Metab 6:95–104, 1986

Dintenfass L, Zador I: Blood rheology in patients with depressive and schizoid anxiety. Biorheology 13:33–36, 1976

Dintenfass L, Zador I: Hemorheology, chronic anxiety and psychosomatic pain: an apparent link. Lex Scientica 13:154–162, 1977

Duffy E: Activation, in Handbook of Psychophysiology. Edited by Greenfield NS, Sternbach RA. New York, Holt, Rinehart and Winston, 1972, pp 577–622

Edvinsson L: Sympathetic control of cerebral circulation. Trends Neurosci 5:425–429, 1982

Edvinsson L, MacKenzie ET: Amine mechanisms in the cerebral circulation. Pharmacol Rev 28:275–353, 1977

Fontaine R, Brenton G, Dery R, et al: MRI in panic disorder: subcortical atrophy and decreased signal in T_1. Paper presented at the Society of Biological Psychiatry, Chicago, IL, May 1987

Forster A, Juge O, Morel D: Effects of midazolam on cerebral blood flow in human subjects. Anesthesiology 56:453–455, 1982

Frackowiak RSJ: The pathophysiology of human cerebral ischemia: a new perspective obtained with positron tomography. Q J Med 57:713–727, 1985

Frackowiak RSJ: An introduction to positron tomography and its application to clinical investigation, in New Brain Imaging Techniques and Psychopharmacology. British Association for Psychopharmacology Monogr No 9. Edited by Trimble MR. Oxford, UK, Oxford University Press, 1986, pp 25–34

Frankenhaeuser M: Brain and circulating catecholamines. Brain Res 31:241–262, 1971

Frewen TC, Sumabat WO, Del Maestro RF: Cerebral blood flow, metabolic rate and cross-brain oxygen consumption in brain injury. J Pediatr 107:510–513, 1985

Fried R: The Hyperventilation Syndrome: Research and Clinical Treatment. Baltimore, MD, Johns Hopkins University Press, 1987

Fuster JM: The prefrontal cortex, in Anatomy, Physiology and Neuropsychology of the Frontal Lobe. New York, Raven Press, 1980, pp 125–145

Galin D: Implications for psychiatry of left and right hemispheric specialization. Arch Gen Psychiatry 31:572–573, 1974

Gibbs FA, Gibbs EL, Lennox WG: The cerebral blood flow in man as influenced by adrenalin, caffeine, amyl nitrite and histamine. Am Heart J 10:916–924, 1935

Gloor P, Olivier A, Quesney LF, et al: The role of the limbic system in experimental phenomena of temporal lobe epilepsy. Ann Neurol 12:129–144, 1982

Goldman-Rakic PS: The frontal lobes: uncharted provinces of the brain. Trends Neurosci 7:425–429, 1984

Gorman JM: Panic disorders, in Anxiety. Edited by Klein DF. New York, S Karger, 1987, pp 36–90

Gorman JM, Askanaz J, Liebowitz MR, et al: Response to hyperventilation in a group of patients with panic disorder. Am J Psychiatry 141:857–861, 1984

Gotoh F, Meyer JS, Takagi Y: Cerebral effects of hyperventilation in man. Arch Neurol 12:410–423, 1965

Gray JAC: The Neuropsychology of Anxiety: An Enquiry Into the Functions of the Septo-Hippocampal System. New York, Oxford University Press, 1982

Griez E, van den Hout MA: Effects of carbon dioxide inhalation on subjective anxiety and some investigative parameters. J Behav Ther Exp Psychiatry 13:27–32, 1982

Gur RC, Gur RE, Obrist WD, et al: Sex and handedness differences in cerebral blood flow during rest and cognitive activity. Science 217:659–661, 1982

Gur RE, Gur RC, Skolnick BE, et al: Brain function in psychiatric disorders, III: regional cerebral blood flow in unmedicated schizophrenics. Arch Gen Psychiatry 42:329–334, 1985

Gur RC, Gur RE, Resnick SM, et al: The effect of anxiety on cortical cerebral blood flow and metabolism. J Cereb Blood Flow Metab 7:173–177, 1987

Guyton AC: Basic Neuroscience. Philadelphia, PA, WB Saunders, 1987

Halgren E, Walter R: Mental phenomena evoked by electrical stimulation of the human hippocampal formation of the amygdala. Brain 101:83–117, 1978

Harik SI, Sharma VK, Wetherbee JR, et al: Adrenergic and cholinergic receptors of cerebral microvessels. J Cereb Blood Flow Metab 1:329–338, 1981

Hebb DO: Drives and the CNS (conceptual nervous system). Psychol Rev 62:243–254, 1955

Heiss WD, Pawlik G, Herholz K, et al: Regional cerebral glucose metabolism in man during wakefulness, asleep, and dreaming. Brain Res 327:362–366, 1985

Hoehn-Saric R: Neurotransmitters in anxiety. Arch Gen Psychiatry 39:735–742, 1982

Hoffman JM, Guze BH, Hawk TC, et al: Cerebral glucose metabolism in normal individuals: effects of aging, sex, and handedness. Neurology 38 (suppl 1): 371, 1988

Ingvar DH: Hyperfrontal distribution of the cerebral gray matter flow in resting wakefulness: on the functional anatomy of the conscious state. Acta Neurol Scand 60:12–25, 1979

Ingvar DH, Lassen NA: Quantitative determination of cerebral blood flow in man. Lancet 2:806–807, 1961

Ingvar DH, Lassen NA: Regulation of cerebral blood flow, in Brain Metabolism and Cerebral Disorders. Edited by Himueich HE. New York, Spectrum Publications, 1976, pp 181–206

Ingvar DH, Soderberg UMK: A new method for measuring cerebral blood flow in relation to the electroencephalogram. Electroencephalogr Clin Neurophysiol 3:403–412, 1956

Ingvar DH, Soderberg U: Cortical blood flow related to EEG patterns evoked by stimulation of the brain stem. Acta Physiol Scand 42:130–143, 1958

Ingvar DH, Haggendal E, Nilsson NJ, et al: Cerebral circulation and metabolism in a conscious patient. Arch Neurol 11:13–21, 1964

Isaacson RL: The Limbic System. New York, Plenum, 1982

Juge O, Meyer JS, Sakai F, et al: Critical appraisal of cerebral blood flow measured from brain stem and cerebellar regions after [133]xenon inhalation in humans. Stroke 10:428–437, 1979

Kandel ER, Schwartz JH: Principles of Neurological Science. Amsterdam, Elsevier, 1981

Kelly A, Munan L: Hematologic profile of natural populations: red cell parameters. Br J Haematol 35:153–160, 1977

Kelly D: Neurosurgical treatment of psychiatric disorders, in Recent Advances in Clinical Psychiatry, No 2. Edited by Granville-Grossman K. London, Churchill Livingstone, 1976, pp 227–261

Kelly DHW, Walter CJS: The relationship between clinical diagnosis and anxiety, assessed by forearm blood flow and other measurements. Br J Psychiatry 112:871–882, 1969

Kennedy C, Gillin JC, Mendelson W, et al: Local cerebral glucose utilization in non–rapid eye movement sleep. Nature 297:325–327, 1982

Kety SS: Consciousness and the metabolism of the brain, in Conference on Problems of Consciousness (Third Conference). Edited by Abramson HA. New York, Josiah Macey Foundation, 1952, pp 11–75

Kety SS, Schmidt CF: The nitrous oxide method for the quantitative determination of cerebral blood flow in man: theory, procedure and normal values. J Clin Invest 27:476–483, 1948

King BD, Sokoloff L, Wechsler RL: The effects of l-epinephrine and l-norepinephrine upon cerebral circulation and metabolism in man. J Clin Invest 31:273–279, 1952

Lader M: The Psychophysiology of Mental Illness. London, Routledge & Kegan Paul, 1975

Lader M: Biological differentiation of anxiety, arousal and stress, in The Biology of Anxiety. Edited by Mathew RJ. New York, Brunner/Mazel, 1982, pp 11–22

Lassen NA, Astrup J: Ischemic penumbra, in Cerebral Blood Flow: Physiological and Clinical Aspects. Edited by Wood JH. New York, McGraw-Hill, 1987, pp 458–466

Lasvennes F, Lestage P, Bobillier P, et al: Stress and local cerebral blood flow: studies on restrained and unrestrained rats. Exp Brain Res 63:163–168, 1986

Lawrence JH, Berlin NI: Relative polycythemia—the polycythemia of stress. Yale J Biol Med 24:498–505, 1951

Ledoux JE, Thompson ME, Iadecola C, et al: Local cerebral blood flow increases during auditory and visual processing in the conscious rat. Science 221:576–578, 1983

Levi L: Stress and distress in response to psychosocial stimuli. Acta Medica Scandinavica (Supplement) 528:1–166, 1972

Ley R, Walker H: Effects of carbon dioxide–oxygen inhalation on heart rate, blood pressure and subjective anxiety. J Behav Ther Exp Psychiatry 4:223–228, 1973

Lindsley DB: Emotion, in Handbook of Experimental Psychology. Edited by SS Stevens. New York, Wiley, 1951, pp 473–516

Lindsley DB: The reticular activating system and perceptual integration, in Electrical Stimulation of the Brain. Edited by Skeers DE. Austin, TX, University of Texas Press, 1961, pp 331–349

Luria AR: The Working Brain: An Introduction to Neuropsychology. New York, Basic Books, 1973

Malmo RB: Activation: a neuropsychological dimension. Psychol Rev 66:367–386, 1959

Mamo H, Meric P, Luft A, et al: Hyperfrontal pattern of human cerebral circulation: variations with age and atherosclerotic state. Arch Neurol 40:626–632, 1983

Marshall J: The viscosity factor in cerebral ischaemia. J Cereb Blood Flow Metabol 2 (suppl 1):S47–S49, 1982

Mathew RJ: Hyperfrontality of regional cerebral blood flow distribution in normals during resting wakefulness: fact or artifact. Biol Psychiatry 26:717–724, 1989

Mathew RJ, Wilson WH: Caffeine induced changes in cerebral circulation. Stroke 16:814–817, 1985

Mathew RJ, Wilson WH: Hematocrit and anxiety. J Psychosom Res 30:307–311, 1986

Mathew RJ, Wilson WH: Elevated hematocrit in patients with schizophrenia. Biol Psychiatry 22:907–910, 1987

Mathew RJ, Wilson WH: Cerebral blood flow changes induced by CO_2 in anxiety. Psychiatry Res 23:285–294, 1988

Mathew RJ, Wilson WH: Cerebral blood flow responses to CO_2 and acetazolamide: the effect of anxiety. Psychiatry Res 28:241–242, 1989a

Mathew RJ, Wilson WH: Epinephrine-induced anxiety and regional cerebral blood flow in anxious patients, in New Directions in Affective Disorders. Edited by Lerer B, Gershon S. New York, Springer-Verlag, 1989b, pp 401–403

Mathew RJ, Wilson WH: Behavioral and cerebrovascular effects of caffeine in patients with anxiety disorders. Acta Psychiatr Scand 82:17–22, 1990

Mathew RJ, Ho BT, Francis DJ, et al: Catecholamines and anxiety. Acta Psychiatr Scand 65:142–147, 1982a

Mathew RJ, Weinman ML, Claghorn JL: Anxiety and cerebral blood flow, in The Biology of Anxiety. Edited by Mathew RJ. New York, Brunner/Mazel, 1982b, pp 23–33

Mathew RJ, Barr DL, Weinman ML: Caffeine and cerebral blood flow. Br J Psychiatry 143:604–608, 1983

Mathew RJ, Margolin RA, Kessler RM: Cerebral function, blood flow, and metabolism: a new vista in psychiatric research. Integrative Psychiatry 3:214–225, 1985a

Mathew RJ, Wilson WH, Daniel DG: The effect of non-sedating doses of diazepam on regional cerebral blood flow. Biol Psychiatry 20:1109–1116, 1985b

Mathew RJ, Wilson WH, Tant SR: Determinants of resting regional cerebral blood flow in normal subjects. Biol Psychiatry 21:907–914, 1986

Mathew RJ, Wilson WH, Nicassio PM: Cerebral ischemic symptoms in anxiety disorders. Am J Psychiatry 144:265, 1987

Mathew RJ, Wilson WH, Tant S: Acute changes in cerebral blood flow associated with marijuana smoking. Acta Psychiatr Scand 79:118–128, 1989a

Mathew RJ, Wilson WH, Tant S: Response to hypercarbia induced by acetazolamide in panic disorder patients. Am J Psychiatry 146:996–1000, 1989b

Maximilian VA, Prohovnik I, Risberg J: Cerebral hemodynamic response to mental activation in normo- and hypercapnia. Stroke 11:342–347, 1980

Mazziotta JC: PET scanning: principles and applications. Discussions in Neurosciences 2(1):9–47, 1985

Mazziotta JC, Phelps ME, Miller J, et al: Tomographic mapping of human cerebral metabolism: normal unstimulated state. Neurology 31:503–516, 1981

Mazziotta JC, Phelps ME, Carson RE, et al: Tomographic mapping of human cerebral metabolism: sensory deprivation. Ann Neurol 12:435–444, 1982

McNair DM, Lorr M, Doppleman LF: Manual for Profile of Mood States. San Diego, CA, Educational and Industrial Testing Service, 1971

Menon D, Koles Z, Dobbs A: The relationship between cerebral blood flow and the EEG in normals. Can J Neurol Sci 7:195–198, 1980

Mesulam MM, Mufson EJ: Insula of the old world monkey, I: architectonics in the insula-orbito-temporal component of the paralimbic brain. J Comp Neurol 212:1–22, 1982

Metter EJ, Riege WH, Kuhl DE, et al: Cerebral metabolic relationships for selected brain regions in healthy adults. J Cereb Blood Flow Metab 4:1–7, 1984

Meyer JS, Ishihara N, Deshmukh VD, et al: Improved method for non-invasive measurement of regional cerebral blood flow by [133]xenon inhalation, Part I: description of method and normal values obtained in healthy volunteers. Stroke 9:195–205, 1978

Meyer JS, Heyman A, Amano T, et al: Mapping local blood flow of human brain by CT scanning during stable xenon inhalation. Stroke 12:426–436, 1981

Moran MA, Mufson EJ, Mesulam MM: Neural inputs into the temporopolar cortex of the rhesus monkey. J Comp Neurol 256:88–103, 1987

Morrow GR, Labrum AH: The relationship between psychological and physiological measures of anxiety. Psychol Med 8:95–101, 1978

Moruzzi G, Magoun HW: Brain stem reticular formation and activation of the EEG. Electroencephalogr Clin Neurophysiol 1:455–473, 1949

Mountz JM, Modell JG, Wilson MW, et al: Positron emission tomographic evaluation of cerebral blood flow during state anxiety in simple phobia. Arch Gen Psychiatry 46:501–504, 1989

Nahas GG, Harvey DJ, Paris M, et al: Marijuana in Science and Medicine. New York, Raven Press, 1984

Nauta WJH: The problem of frontal lobe: a reinterpretation. J Psychiatr Res 8:167–187, 1971

Nesse RM, Cameron OG, Curtis GC, et al: Adrenergic function in patients with panic anxiety. Arch Gen Psychiatry 41:771–776, 1984

Noback CR: The Human Nervous System: Basic Principles of Neurobiology, 2nd Edition. New York, McGraw-Hill, 1975

Nordahl TE, Benkelfat C, Semple WE, et al: Cerebral glucose metabolic rates in obsessive-compulsive disorder. Neuropsychopharmacology 2:23–28, 1989

Nordahl TE, Semple WE, Gross M, et al: Cerebral glucose metabolic differences in patients with panic disorder. Neuropsychopharmacology 3:261–272, 1990

Obrist WD, Thompson HK, Wang HS, et al: Regional cerebral blood flow estimated by [133]xenon inhalation. Stroke 6:245–256, 1975

Obrist WD, Gennarelli TA, Segawa H, et al: Relation of cerebral blood flow to neurological status and outcome in head-injured patients. J Neurosurg 51:292–300, 1979

Ohata M, Fredricks WR, Sunderan U, et al: Effects of immobilization stress on regional cerebral blood flow in the conscious rat. J Cereb Blood Flow Metab 1:187–194, 1984

Olesen J: Effect of intracarotid isoprenaline, propranolol, and prostaglandin E on regional cerebral blood flow in man, in Blood Flow and Metabolism in the Brain. Edited by Harper M, Jennett B, Miller D, et al. London, Churchill Livingstone, 1975, pp 4.10–4.11

Olesen J, Paulson B, Lassen NA: Regional cerebral blood flow in man determined by the initial slope of the clearance of intra-arterially injected [133]xenon. Stroke 2:519–540, 1971

Pitts FN, Allen RE: Beta-adrenergic blockade in the treatment of anxiety, in The Biology of Anxiety. Edited by Mathew RJ. New York, Brunner/Mazel, 1982, pp 134–161

Powers WJ, Raichle ME: Positron emission tomography and its application to the study of cerebrovascular disease in man. Stroke 16:361–376, 1986

Pribram KH: The primate frontal cortex: executive of the brain, in Psychophysiology of the Frontal Lobes. Edited by Pribram KH, Luria AR. New York, Academic, 1973, pp 293–314

Price RR, Patton JA, Rollo FD: Single photon emission computed tomography: an overview, in Single Photon Emission Computed Tomography and Other Selected Computer Topics. Edited by Sorenson JA. New York, The Society of Nuclear Medicine, 1980, pp 1–18

Prohovnik I: Cerebral lateralization of psychologic processes: a literature review. Arch Psychol (Frankf) 130:S161–S211, 1978

Prohovnik I, Hakansson K, Risberg J: Observations on the functional significance of regional cerebral blood flow in resting normal subjects. Neuropsychologia 18:203–217, 1980

Purves MJ: The Physiology of Cerebral Circulation. Cambridge, UK, Cambridge University Press, 1972

Raichle M, Grubb RL, Gado MH, et al: Correlation between regional cerebral blood flow and oxidative metabolism: in vivo studies in man. Arch Neurol 33:523–526, 1976

Rapoport SI, Ohata M, Sundaram U, et al: Regional cerebral blood flow following immobilization stress in the conscious rat. J Cereb Blood Flow Metab 1:477–478, 1981

Rapoport SI, Duara D, Grady CL, et al: Cerebral glucose utilization in relation to age in man, in The Metabolism of the Human Brain Studied With Positron Emission Tomography. Edited by Greitz T, Ingvar DH, Widen L. New York, Raven, 1985, pp 339–350

Reiman EM: PET, panic disorder, and normal anticipatory anxiety, in Neurobiology of Panic Disorder. (Frontiers of Clinical Neuroscience, Vol 8.) Edited by Ballenger JC. New York, Wiley–AR Liss, 1990, pp 245–270

Reiman EM, Raichle ME, Butler FK, et al: A focal brain abnormality in panic disorder, a severe form of anxiety. Nature 310:683–685, 1984

Reiman EM, Raichle ME, Robins E, et al: The application of positron emission tomography to the study of panic disorder. Am J Psychiatry 143:469–477, 1986

Reiman EM, Fusselman MJ, Fox BJ, et al: Neuroanatomical correlates of anticipatory anxiety. Science 243:1071–1074, 1989a

Reiman EM, Raichle ME, Robins E, et al: Neuroanatomical correlates of a lactate-induced anxiety attack. Arch Gen Psychiatry 46:493–500, 1989b

Reivich M, Gur R, Alavi A: Positron emission tomographic studies of sensory stimuli, cognitive processes and anxiety. Human Neurobiology 2:25–33, 1983

Risberg J, Maximilian AV, Prohovnik I: Changes in cortical activity patterns during habituation to a reasoning test. Neuropsychologia 15:793–798, 1977

Risberg J, Gustafson L, Prohovnik I: rCBF measurements by [133]xenon inhalation: applications in neuropsychology and psychiatry. Progress in Nuclear Medicine 7:82–94, 1981

Rockoff MA, Naughton KVH, Shapiro HM, et al: Cerebral circulatory and metabolic responses to intravenously administered lorazepam. Anesthesiology 53:215–218, 1980

Rodriguez G, Cogorno P, Gris A, et al: Regional cerebral blood flow and anxiety: a correlational study in neurologically normal patients. J Cereb Blood Flow Metab 9:410–416, 1989

Rosenblum WI, Guilianti D: Participation of cerebrovascular nerves in generalized sympathetic discharge. Arch Neurol 29:91–94, 1973

Ross ED: Right hemisphere's role in language, affecture behavior and emotion. Trends Neurosci 7:342–346, 1984

Routtenberg A: The two arousal hypothesis: reticular formation and the limbic systems. Psychol Rev 75:51–80, 1968

Russell RP, Conley CL: Benign polycythemia: Gaisbock's syndrome. Arch Intern Med 114:734–740, 1964

Sakai F, Meyer JS, Yamaguchi F, et al: [133]Xenon inhalation method for measuring cerebral blood flow in conscious baboons. Stroke 10:310–318, 1979

Sakai F, Meyer JS, Karacan I, et al: Normal human sleep: regional cerebral hemodynamics. Ann Neurol 7:471–478, 1980

Sarason IG: Stress, anxiety and cognitive interference: reaction to tests. J Pers Soc Psychol 46:929–938, 1984

Schachter S, Singer JE: Cognitive social and physiological determinants of emotional state. Psychol Rev 69:379–399, 1962

Schildkraut JJ, Kety SS: Biogenic amines and emotion. Science 156:21–30, 1967

Selye H: The Stress of Life, New York, McGraw-Hill, 1956

Sensenbach W, Madison L, Ochs L: A comparison of the effects of l-norepinephrine, synthetic l-epinephrine, and USP-epinephrine upon cerebral blood flow and metabolism in man. J Clin Invest 32:226–232, 1953

Shakhnovich AR, Serbinenko FA, Razumovsky A Ye, et al: The dependence of cerebral blood flow on mental activity and on emotional state in man. Neuropsychologia 18:465–476, 1980

Sharma HS, Dey PK: Influence of long-term immobilization stress on regional blood-brain barrier permeability, cerebral blood flow and 5-HT level in conscious normotensive young rats. J Neurol Sci 72:61–76, 1986

Siegel JM: Behavioral functions of the reticular formation. Brain Res 180:69–105, 1979

Siesjo BK: Cerebral metabolic rate in hypercarbia—a controversy. Journal of Anesthesiology 52:461–465, 1980

Sokoloff L, Mangold R, Wechsler R, et al: The effect of mental arithmetic on cerebral blood flow and metabolism. J Clin Invest 34:1101–1108, 1955

Spielberger CD, Gorsuch RL, Lushene RD: State-Trait Anxiety Inventory Manual. Palo Alto, CA, Consulting Psychologists Press, 1970

Stewart RS, Devous MD, Rush AJ, et al: Cerebral blood flow changes during sodium-lactate induced panic attacks. Am J Psychiatry 145:442–449, 1988

Strandgaard S, Paulson OB: Cerebral autoregulation. Stroke 15:413–416, 1984

Stuss DT, Benson DF: The Frontal Lobes. New York, Raven, 1986

Swedo SE, Schapiro MB, Grady CL, et al: Cerebral glucose metabolism in childhood-onset obsessive-compulsive disorder. Arch Gen Psychiatry 46:518–523, 1989

Thomas DJ: Whole blood viscosity and cerebral blood flow. Stroke 13:285–287, 1982

Townsend RE, Prinz PN, Obrist WD: Human cerebral blood flow during sleep and waking. J Appl Physiol 35:620–625, 1973

Tucker DM, Roth RS, Arneson BA, et al: Right hemispheric activation during stress. Neuropsychologia 15:697–700, 1977

Tucker DM, Antes JR, Stenslie CE, et al: Anxiety and lateral cerebral function. J Abnorm Psychol 87:380–383, 1978

Tyler SK, Tucker DM: Anxiety and perceptual structure: individual differences in neuropsychological function. J Abnorm Psychol 91:210–220, 1982

Tyrer P: The Role of Bodily Feelings in Anxiety. London, Oxford University Press, 1976

van den Hout MA, Griez E: Panic symptoms after the inhalation of carbon dioxide. Br J Psychiatry 144:503–507, 1984

Veleber DM, Templer DI: Effects of caffeine on anxiety and depression. J Abnorm Psychol 93:120–122, 1984

Vernheit J, Renou AM, Orgogozo JM, et al: Effects of a diazepam-fentanyl mixture on cerebral blood flow and oxygen consumption in man. Br J Anaesth 50:165–169, 1978

Wall M, Mielke D, Luther JS: Panic attacks and psychomotor seizures following right temple labectomy. J Clin Psychiatry 47:219, 1986

Warach S, Gur RC, Gur RE, et al: The reproducibility of the [133]Xenon inhalation technique in resting studies: task order and sex related effects in healthy young adults. J Cereb Blood Flow Metab 7:702–708, 1987

Weil AT: Adverse reactions to marijuana. N Engl J Med 282:997–1000, 1970

Weinberger DR, Berman KF, Zec RF: Physiologic dysfunction of dorso-lateral prefrontal cortex in schizophrenia, I: regional cerebral blood flow evidence. Arch Gen Psychiatry 43:114–124, 1986

Wilkinson IMS, Bull JWD, Du Boulay GH, et al: Regional blood flow in normal cerebral hemisphere. J Neurol Neurosurg Psychiatry 32:367–378, 1969

Wilson SJ, Boyle P: Erroneous anaemea and polycythemia. Arch Intern Med 90:602–609, 1952

Woods SW, Charney DS, Goodman WK, et al: Carbon dioxide sensitivity in panic anxiety: ventilatory and anxiogenic response to carbon dioxide in healthy subjects and patients with panic anxiety before and after alprazolam treatment. Arch Gen Psychiatry 43:900–909, 1986

Woods SW, Koster K, Krystal JK, et al: Yohimbine alters regional cerebral blood flow in panic disorder. Lancet 2:678, 1988

Yoshii F, Barker WW, Chang JY, et al: Sensitivity of cerebral glucose metabolism to age, gender, brain volume, brain atrophy, and cerebro-vascular risk factors. J Cereb Blood Flow Metab 8:654–661, 1988

Zohar J, Insel TR, Berman KF, et al: Anxiety and cerebral blood flow during behavioral challenge: dissociation of central from peripheral and subjective measures. Arch Gen Psychiatry 46:505–510, 1989

Chapter 2

Serotonin in the Pathogenesis of Anxiety

René S. Kahn, M.D., and Clare Moore, M.S.

U ntil recently, most studies examining a possible role for serotonin (5-hydroxytryptamine [5-HT]) in psychopathology focused on depressive disorders and aggression. However, in recent years there has been an explosive growth of studies examining a possible role of 5-HT dysfunction in the pathogenesis of anxiety. Specifically, abnormal 5-HT function has been suggested to be involved in the pathogenesis of obsessive-compulsive disorder (OCD) (Zohar and Insel 1987), panic disorder (Kahn and van Praag 1988), and generalized anxiety disorder (GAD) (Kahn et al. 1988b). In this chapter we will review the role of 5-HT in the pathogenesis of these anxiety disorders.

Although a role for 5-HT in anxiety has only recently become the focus of study in human subjects, a substantial body of animal work has indicated that 5-HT and anxiety are related. It is worth noting that as the interest in a role for 5-HT in human forms of anxiety has expanded, the number of studies examining the effect of 5-HT on anxiety in animals has also increased. We will first review the compelling evidence from animal studies suggesting a role for 5-HT in anxiety before venturing into a review of human studies.

ANATOMY AND PHYSIOLOGY OF SEROTONIN IN THE BRAIN

In contrast to their widespread projections, the cell bodies of 5-HT–producing neurons are rather discretely localized in the dorsal and medial raphe nuclei of the brain stem. From these nuclei six major projections ascend to the forebrain; two tracts within the median forebrain bundle and four outside it. The targets of these projections include the cortex, hypothalamus, thalamus, basal ganglia, substantia nigra, caudate, putamen, amygdala, hippocampus, septum, tegmentum, and mammillary bodies (Azmitia and Segal 1978).

Three major subcategories of 5-HT receptors have been identified in the central nervous system (CNS) and are designated 5-HT_1, 5-HT_2, and 5-HT_3. 5-HT_1 receptors have been further classified as 5-HT_{1A}, 5-HT_{1B}, 5-HT_{1C}, and 5-HT_{1D} subtypes. 5-HT_{1A} receptors are found in the frontal cortex and hippocampus of the human brain (Hoyer et al. 1986a) and are located presynaptically as autoreceptors (and as such inhibit intrinsic raphe firing [Trulson and Arasteh 1985]), in addition to being located postsynaptically. Stimulation of these receptors has been reported to activate adenylate cyclase (Hoyer 1988). In the rat, stimulation of the 5-HT_{1A} receptor induces the release of adrenocorticotropin (ACTH) (Gilbert et al. 1988) and prolactin (Willoughby et al. 1988), and decreases body temperature and food intake (Aulakh et al. 1988). The 5-HT_{1A} receptor was recently cloned (Fargin et al. 1988). 5-HT_{1B} receptors have not been found in human brain. 5-HT_{1C} receptors, however, have been found in the choroid plexus and cortex (Hoyer et al. 1986b) and reportedly increase phosphatidyl turnover (Conn et al. 1986). These receptors have also been cloned (Julius et al. 1988) and have shown a 51% homology with the 5-HT_2 receptor (Pritchett et al. 1988). This structural similarity explains the functional overlap between 5-HT_{1C} and 5-HT_2 receptors. Both receptors increase phosphatidyl turnover when stimulated. Additionally, antagonists to 5-HT_2 receptors show approximately equal affinity to 5-HT_{1C} receptors (Sanders-Bush and Breeding 1988). Moreover, it has even been suggested that the 5-HT_{1C} receptor should be reclassified as a 5-HT_2 subreceptor because it shows better homology with the 5-HT_2 receptor than with the 5-HT_{1A} receptor. (Only 35% homology has been found between the 5-HT_{1C} and 5-HT_{1A} receptors [Pritchett et al. 1988].)

The 5-HT_{1D} receptor appears to be the predominant type of 5-HT_1 binding site in bovine brain (Heuring and Peroutka 1987), and it also has been found in the human cortex, caudate, and substantia nigra (Waeber et al. 1988). It has been suggested that the 5-HT$_{1D}$ may be the human equivalent of the 5-HT$_{1B}$ receptor found in other animals (Hoyer 1988). In contrast to the 5-HT$_{1A}$ receptor, the 5-HT$_{1D}$ receptor appears to be negatively coupled to adenylate cyclase (Schoeffter et al. 1988), but its functional effects remain unclear.

5-HT$_2$ receptors are particularly abundant in the hippocampus and frontal cortex in both animals and humans (Hoyer et al. 1986b) and are, as already stated, linked to phosphatidyl turnover. Stimulation of 5-HT$_2$ receptors has been found to cause various peripheral effects such as platelet aggregation (Hoyer 1988). Its central effects, however, are far less well known.

By specific labeling with experimental drugs (i.e., GR 38032, GR 65630, and BRL 43694), the 5-HT$_3$ receptors have been found to be located in the cortex and limbic areas of the rat brain (Kilpatrick et al. 1987).

ANIMAL EXPERIMENTS

Methodological Issues

In animal laboratory studies of anxiety the major methodological problem is that emotion must be inferred from observable behavioral changes. Several paradigms frequently used to operationalize the construct of anxiety in animals have been 1) introduction of a conflict situation, 2) exposure to novel stimuli, and 3) use of the X-maze.

The *conflict paradigm* is based on a conditioned emotional response (CER) model (Estes and Skinner 1941). In this model the animal is conditioned to press a bar in order to obtain a reward, usually food. Later, a signal such as a bright light is introduced following bar pressing, coupled with a punishment such as an electric shock. The animal faced with the conflict situation between reward and punishment decreases its bar pressing. This "behavioral suppression" is taken to be the result of anxiety.

The *novel environment model* involves placing the animal in a large, ceilingless, brightly lit box. In this situation animals tend to show decreased exploratory behavior (Crawley and Goodwin

1980) and decreased social interaction (File 1985), both of which are regarded as indicators of anxiety.

The *X-maze (or elevated plus-maze) anxiety model* is a modification of the novel environment model that involves a maze with open and enclosed arms. General motor inhibition is expressed as a decrease in entries into both open and enclosed arms, while increased anxiety without generalized motor inhibition results in decreased entries only into the open arms of the X-maze. Anxiolytic effects are reflected by increased entries into the open arms of the maze (Montgomery 1955). A major advantage of the X-maze model is that it can be used to measure both increased and decreased anxiety. The unmodified novel environment model and the conflict model are unable to assess increased anxiety in the animal because it is not possible to distinguish generalized motor inhibition from anxiety-induced motor inhibition.

Manipulation of the Serotonergic System

In order to assess the possible relationship between 5-HT function and anxiety in animals, studies have been carried out measuring animal anxiety equivalents while manipulating 5-HT function.

Decrease of Serotonin Function

Inhibition of serotonin synthesis.   One method of reducing 5-HT function is to inhibit 5-HT synthesis altogether. By utilizing *p*-chlorophenylalanine (p-CPA), a 5-HT synthesis inhibitor, 5-HT availability can be decreased by about 90%. It should be noted, though, that p-CPA also has a slight effect (depending on the dose) on the availability of norepinephrine. As Table 2–1 indicates, p-CPA consistently causes release from behavioral suppression in animal anxiety models. This effect is abolished by the administration of 5-hydroxytryptophan (5-HTP) (Engel et al. 1984; Geller and Blum 1970; Stein et al. 1973; Tye et al. 1979) or the 5-HT$_{1A}$ agonists 5-methoxy-dimethyltryptamine (5-MeO-DMT) (Shephard et al. 1982) and 8-hydroxy-2-(di-*n*-propylamino) tetralin (8-OH-DPAT) (Engel et al. 1984). Augmentation of dopamine and norepinephrine function through administration of

Table 2–1. Animal studies: decrease of serotonin function using p-chlorophenylalanine

Author(s)	Model[a]	Effect	Comment[b]
Robichaud and Sledge 1969	G + S	Release of suppression	
Geller and Blum 1970	G + S	Release of suppression	Reversed by 5-HTP
Wise et al. 1972	G + S	Release of suppression	
Blakely and Parker 1973	G + S	No effect	
Stein et al. 1973	G + S	Release of suppression	Reversed by 5-HTP
Tye et al. 1977	G + S	Release of suppression	Reversed by 5-HTP not dopa
Shephard et al.1982	G + S	Release of suppression	Reversed by 5-MeO-DMT
Engel et al.1984	G + S	Release of suppression	Reversed by 5-HTP, 8-OH-DPAT
Kilts et al. 1981	Water-lick	Release of suppression	
Petersen and Lassen 1981	Water-lick	Release of suppression	
Ellison 1977	NE	Release of inhibition	
File and Hyde 1977	NE	Release of inhibition	

[a]G + S = Geller and Seifter model (Geller and Seifter 1960) and related models; water-lick = water-lick model (Vogel et al. 1971); NE = Novel environment (File 1985) and related models.
[b]5-HTP = 5-hydroxytryptophan; dopa = deoxyphenylalanine; 5-MeO-DMT = 5=methoxy-dimethyltryptamine; 8-OH-DPAT = 8-hydroxy-2(di-n-propylamino)tetralin.

dopa, the precursor of both dopamine and noradenaline, does not reverse the p-CPA effect (Tye et al. 1979), suggesting that catecholamines are not involved in p-CPA's anxiolytic effects.

The objection might be raised that the anxiolytic effects of p-CPA are mediated by behavioral mechanisms other than anxiety reduction because p-CPA directly increases food intake (Blundell 1984) and drinking (Barofski et al. 1980). Because conflict-based anxiety models depend on food and water as positive reinforcers, one might argue that p-CPA's effects are secondary to the direct stimulation of food intake and not to decreased anxiety. It seems more likely, however, that p-CPA is anxiolytic, because its effects are observed in the novel environment model, which does not depend on a food or water reward.

Destruction of serotonin neurons.   Another method of reducing 5-HT function is the use of agents toxic to 5-HT neurons. Both 5,7-dihydroxytryptamine (DHT) and 5,6-DHT eliminate 5-HT neurons in specific brain regions. In several studies the localized destruction of regions containing 5-HT resulted in diminished anxiety responses. In the Geller and Seifter (1960) model, injection of DHT into the ventral tegmentum produced a marked release from behavioral suppression 11 days after administration (Tye et al. 1977). A similar effect was demonstrated following intraventricular DHT administration in the *water-lick model* (Lippa et al. 1979), and also in a more recent study using the X-maze animal anxiety model (Briley et al. 1990). In this latter study, rats showed increased entries into the open (but not closed) arms in the X-maze 14 days after intracerebroventricular DHT administration, which suggests that DHT has anxiolytic effects (Briley et al. 1990). In a novel environment model, DHT lesioning of the dorsal raphe resulted in anxiety reduction 12 days later, whereas lesions to the median raphe did not result in the same reduction (File et al. 1979). The latter findings suggest functional specificity for different 5-HT anatomic regions and possibly a greater involvement of the dorsal raphe systems in anxiety mechanisms. In addition, anxiolytic effects were observed 14 days after lateral septum lesioning. In contrast, also in a novel environment model, no anxiety reduction was found after destruction of catecholamine neurons with 6-hydroxydopamine, suggesting that catecholaminergic systems were not involved (Clarke and File 1982).

Assessing the effects of DHT at time points other than the ones used in the above studies has led to varying findings. No anxiety reduction was observed 21 days after intraventricular DHT lesioning in a conflict model (Thiebot et al. 1982), or 3 to 5 days after intraventricular administration in a water-lick model (Commissaris et al. 1981). However, as discussed above, anxiety reduction at 10 to 14 days after DHT administration was shown in several studies. Conceivably, these disparities might be related to differential temporal 5-HT availability, but further investigation is required to clarify this issue.

Serotonin antagonists.   Finally, 5-HT function can be decreased using 5-HT receptor antagonists such as the $5\text{-HT}_{1/2}$ antagonists methysergide, cinanserin, cyproheptadine, and metergoline; the selective $5\text{-HT}_{1C/2}$ antagonist ritanserin; and the 5-HT_3 antagonists GR 38242F and BRL 43694 (Table 2–2). The most consistent finding has been obtained from studies using methysergide in the Geller and Seifter model and 5-HT_3 antagonists in the novel environment model. In contrast, studies using cyproheptadine failed to show consistent anxiety reduction, and the findings with metergoline and cinanserin have been contradictory, though only a small number of studies were conducted.

In a food-motivated punishment model, ritanserin did not reduce anxiety (Colpaert et al. 1985), nor did it have anxiolytic effects in a social interaction model (Gardner 1986). It did, however, have anxiolytic effects in the X-maze model (Critchley and Handley 1987; Pellow et al. 1987).

The selective 5-HT_3 antagonists GR 38032F, BRL 43694, and ICS 205930 had anxiolytic effects in rats (as well as in monkeys [Jones et al. 1987]) in the novel environment model (Costall et al. 1987; Jones et al. 1987; Papp 1988). Piper et al. (1987) also found these agents to have anxiolytic effects in rats in the novel environment model but no effects in rats in the Geller and Seifter model and only weak anxiolytic effects in monkeys.

Interpretation of these findings is hampered by the fact that most of the agents used are not purely selective for 5-HT. Both methysergide and metergoline have pronounced dopaminergic

Table 2–2. Animal studies: decrease of serotonin function using serotonin antagonists

Author	Drug	Dose (mg/kg)	Model[a]	Effect
Graeff and Schoenfeld 1970	Methysergide	0.3	CER	Release of suppression
Winter 1972	Methysergide	3–10	G + S	Release of suppression
Stein et al. 1975	Methysergide	10	G + S	Release of suppression
Graeff 1974	Methysergide	3–10	G + S	Release of suppression
Cook and Sepinwall 1975	Methysergide	1–10	G + S	Release of suppression
Petersen and Lassen 1981	Methysergide	0.3–3.0	Water-lick	Release of suppression
Kilts et al. 1981	Methysergide	1–18	Water-lick	Release of suppression
Gardner 1985	Methysergide	2–20	Water-lick	Release of suppression
Geller et al. 1974	Cinanserin	60	G + S	Release of suppression
Winter 1972	Cinanserin	3–15	G + S	No effect
Sepinwall and Cook 1978	Cinanserin	60	G + S	No effect
Cook and Sepinwall 1975	Cinanserin	15	G + S	Release of suppression
Kilts et al. 1981	Cinanserin	56	Water-lick	Release of suppression
Petersen and Lassen 1981	Cinanserin	10–60	Water-lick	No effect
Petersen and Lassen 1981	Cyproheptadine	1–10	Water-lick	No effect
Kilts et al. 1981	Cyproheptadine	1–18	Water-lick	No effect

Reference	Drug	Dose	Model	Effect
Gardner 1985	Cyproheptadine	10	CER	No effect
Leone et al. 1983	Metergoline	0.3–3.0	CER	Release of suppression
Gardner 1985	Metergoline	10, 20	CER	No effect
Commissaris and Rech 1982	Metergoline	0.25–2.0	Water-lick	No effect
Colpaert et al. 1985	Ritanserin	0.005–5.0	G + S	No effect
Gardner 1986	Ritanserin	0.025–5.0	NE	No effect
Pellow et al. 1987	Ritanserin	0.025–10.0	X-maze	Open arm entries ↑
Critchley and Handley 1987	Ritanserin	0.025–5.0	X-maze	Open arm entries ↑
Costall et al. 1987	GR 38032F	0.005–10.0	NE	Release of inhibition
Costall et al. 1987	BRL 43694	0.001–1.0	NE	Release of inhibition
Jones et al. 1987	GR 38032F	0.01, 0.1	NE	Release of inhibition
Piper et al. 1987	GR 38032F	0.005–5.0	NE	Release of inhibition
Piper et al. 1987	BRL 43694	0.005–5.0	NE	Release of inhibition
Piper et al. 1987	GR 38032F	0.005–5.0	G + S	No effect
Piper et al. 1987	BRL 43694	0.005–5.0	G + S	No effect
Papp 1988	ICS 205930	0.125–1.0	NE	Release of inhibition

[a]CER = conditioned emotional response model (Estes and Skinner 1941); G + S = Geller and Seifter model (Geller and Seifter 1960) and related models; X-maze = X-maze anxiety model (Montgomery 1955).

agonistic effects in doses over 0.1 mg/kg (Krulich et al. 1981). Similarly, cyproheptadine has effects on histamine and choline receptors (Remy et al. 1977). More selective agents (e.g., 5-HT$_2$ and 5-HT$_3$ antagonists have also provided mixed results that may be due to the choice of anxiety models. 5-HT$_3$ antagonists are anxiolytic when tested in the novel environment model, and 5-HT$_2$ antagonists may be anxiolytic when tested in the X-maze model.

Increase of Serotonin Function

Because diminishing 5-HT function results in anxiety reduction, one might predict that increasing 5-HT availability would cause the opposite effect. The results of several studies with a variety of 5-HT agonists leave little doubt that increasing 5-HT function in animals does cause behavioral suppression (see Table 2–3). For example, Graeff and Schoenfeld (1970), using the 5-HT agonist α-methyltryptamine in the basic CER paradigm, reported inhibition of both punished and unpunished responses in pigeons. Similar results were found by Stein et al. (1973) and by Winter (1972) in rats treated with the same agent and with other 5-HT agonists, such as m-chlorophenylpiperazine (m-CPP), fenfluramine (Kilts et al. 1982), and 5-MeO-DMT (Shephard et al. 1982). However, a problem arises when attempting to determine the cause of the behavioral inhibition, because increased 5-HT function is also associated with generalized motor inhibition. Consequently, in these models, 5-HT–induced anxiogenic effects cannot be differentiated from the general effects of 5-HT on motor behavior.

It does appear, however, that the X-maze model can be used to differentiate between anxiogenic and general effects, as stated earlier (Montgomery 1955). In this model the 5-HT$_{1A}$ agonists 8-OH-DPAT and 5-MeO-DMT did in fact selectively decrease open-arm entries of rats, indicating that anxiogenesis had occurred (Critchley and Handley 1987). Similarly, when m-CPP was administered in a social interaction model, which is able to differentiate between nonspecific inhibition (decrease in motor activity) and increased anxiety (decreased social interaction), it was found that it selectively decreased social interaction

(Whitton and Curzon 1990). m-CPP also decreased the number of entries into the open arms of the X-maze in another study (Benjamin et al. 1990). The effects of m-CPP in the social interaction model were blocked by 5-HT$_{1C}$ and 5-HT$_3$ antagonists but not by selective 5-HT$_{1A}$ and 5-HT$_2$ antagonists (Kennett et al. 1989), suggesting that increasing 5-HT function is anxiogenic at the 5-HT$_{1C}$ and 5-HT$_3$ receptors but not at the other 5-HT receptors.

Conclusion: Serotonin and Anxiety in Animals

Decreasing 5-HT function, particularly when the synthesis of 5-HT is blocked, has anxiolytic effects in rodents. Less consistent data have been obtained when 5-HT function is diminished using destruction of 5-HT neurons or when 5-HT antagonists are used. When 5-HT function is increased, it appears to be anxiogenic in animals.

But which, if any, of the multiple 5-HT receptors is involved in the regulation of anxiety? In the animal anxiety studies, decreasing 5-HT function with antagonists selective for one particular 5-HT receptor has produced conflicting results but suggests that the blockade of 5-HT$_{1C/2}$ and 5-HT$_3$ receptors is anxiolytic. The few studies examining the effects of increased 5-HT function in animals may be more informative. They suggest that increasing function at the 5-HT$_{1C}$ and/or 5-HT$_3$ receptor may be anxiogenic. Thus, the very preliminary conclusion may be made that the 5-HT$_{1C/2}$ and 5-HT$_3$ systems are involved in anxiety in animals.

HUMAN EXPERIMENTS

Serotonin and Anxiety in Humans

Assessment of Serotonin Function in Humans

A variety of methods have been used to assess different aspects of 5-HT function in human anxiety studies. These have included studies measuring 5-HT metabolism, challenge studies with 5-HT agonists, and treatment studies with agents altering 5-HT availability.

The most informative method for assessing central 5-HT metabolism is the measurement of the 5-HT metabolite 5-hydroxy-

Table 2-3. Animal studies: increase of serotonin function

Author	Drug (dose)[a]	Model[b]	Effect[c]	Antagonized by[d]	Effect of antagonist
Graeff and Schoenfeld (1970)	α-Methyltryptophan (0.03–3.0 mg/kg im)	CER	Responses ↓		
Winter (1972)	α-Methyltryptophan (0.3–5.0 mg/kg ip)	G + S	Punished resp ↓ Unpunished resp ↓		
Kilts et al. (1982)	m-CPP (1–2 mg/kg ip)	Water-lick	Punished resp ↓ Unpunished resp ↓		
	Fenfluramine (0.25–1.0 mg/kg ip)	Water-lick	No effect No effect		
Shephard et al. (1982)	5-MeO-DMT (1–3 mg/kg ip)	G + S	Punished rep = Unpunished resp ↓		
Critchley and Handley (1987)	8-OH-DPAT (0.015–1.0 mg/kg ip)	X-maze	Open arm entries ↓		
	5-MeO-DMT (0.25–2.5 mg/kg ip)	X-maze	Open arm entries ↓		

Study	Drug (dose)	Model	Result	Antagonist	Effect
Benjamin et al. (1990)	m-CPP (1.5–3.25 mg/kg ip)	X-maze	Open arm entries ↓		
	TFMPP (1.5–3.25 mg/kg ip)		Open arm entries ↓		
Whitton and Curzon (1990)	m-CPP (2–4 µg/kg icv)	NE	SI ↓		
	(1 µg/kg iH)		SI ↓		
	(1 µg/kg iA)		SI =		
Kennet et al. (1989)	m-CPP (0.5 mg/kg ip)	NE	SI ↓	Metergoline (2.5)	Blocked
				Mianserin (2)	Blocked
				Cyproheptadine (2)	Blocked
				Ritanserin (0.6)	No effect
				Ketanserin (0.2)	No effect
				Cyanopindolol (6)	No effect
				Propranolol (16)	No effect
				ICS 205930 (0.05)	Blocked
				ICS 205930 (1)	No effect

Note. ↑/↓ = increase/decrease; "=" indicates no change.

[a] ip = intraperitoneal; icv = intracerebroventricular; iH = in hippocampus; iA = in amygdala; m-CPP = *m*-chlorophenylpiperazine; 5-MeO-DMT = 5-methoxy-dimethyltryptamine; 8-OH-DPAT = 8-hydroxy-2-(di-*n*-propylamino)tetralin; TFMPP = trifluoro-methylphenylpiperazine.

[b] CER = conditioned emotional response model (Estes and Skinner 1941); G + S = Geller and Seifter model (Geller and Seifter 1960) and related models; X-maze = X-maze anxiety model (Montgomery 1955); SI = social interaction; water-lick = water-lick model. (Vogel et al. 1971); NE = novel environment model (File 1985) and related models.

indoleacetic acid (5-HIAA) in cerebrospinal fluid (CSF). Only a few anxiety studies, however, have utilized this method.

Another method, the so-called *challenge paradigm*, is well suited to assessment of central 5-HT receptor sensitivity. However, this method is only valid if the challenge agents, the 5-HT agonists, have high selectivity for the 5-HT receptor (van Praag et al. 1986). Following the administration of a 5-HT agonist, measurement of hormonal and behavioral effects permits an assessment of the state of the central 5-HT receptor system. This method has been utilized in several studies involving panic disorder and OCD patients.

Lastly, treatment studies in anxiety disorders with drugs selective for serotonergic systems have been useful in exploring the relationship between 5-HT and anxiety in humans.

Panic Disorder

Treatment studies.   A number of treatment studies using 5-HT agents in panic disorder suggest that indirect 5-HT agonists are effective antipanic agents. The results of these studies are summarized in Table 2–4. One study compared the effects of L-5-HTP and the 5-HT reuptake inhibitor clomipramine in an 8-week placebo-controlled experiment. Both compounds induced antianxiety and antipanic effects (Kahn et al. 1987). Two subsequent studies examined the efficacy of clomipramine in patients with panic disorder and/or agoraphobia (Cassano et al. 1988; Johnston et al. 1988). The study by Cassano et al. compared the effects of imipramine to those of clomipramine in reducing panic attacks in patients with panic disorder. Although both drugs were equally effective, clomipramine had a faster onset of action (Cassano et al. 1988). In the study by Johnston et al., clomipramine was found to be significantly superior to placebo in reducing both agoraphobic symptoms and panic attacks in female patients suffering from agoraphobia with panic attacks (Johnston et al. 1988).

Attributing the effectiveness of clomipramine solely to serotonergic mechanisms is problematic because its main metabolite, desmethylclomipramine, possesses norepinephrine reuptake–blocking properties, and therefore its therapeutic effects may be mediated through noradrenergic systems. Because the antipanic effects of clomipramine were equivalent to those of fluvoxamine, a selective 5-HT reuptake inhibitor (Den Boer et al. 1987), it is likely that clomipramine's effects are also mediated through the serotonergic system. Moreover, when comparing fluvoxamine to the selective norepinephrine reuptake inhibitor maprotiline, Den Boer and Westenberg (1988) found fluvoxamine to be effective in reducing panic attacks, in contrast to maprotiline. Finally, fluvoxamine was found to be superior to placebo in reducing panic attacks (Den Boer and Westenberg 1990b). Evans et al. (1986) compared zimelidine (also a selective 5-HT reuptake inhibitor) and imipramine in a placebo-controlled study and found zimelidine, but not imipramine, to have antipanic effects. The inefficacy of imipramine in this study is somewhat surprising (see Liebowitz 1985 for a review) and might be related to the small number of patients in the placebo group ($n = 4$). Open pilot studies using other 5-HT agonists such as 5-HTP (Kahn and Westenberg 1985), zimelidine (Evans and Moore 1981; Kokzacks et al. 1981), trazodone (Mavissakalian 1986), and fluoxetine (Gorman et al. 1987) lend further support to the efficacy of 5-HT agonists in panic disorder.

In treatment studies involving indirect 5-HT agonists, an initial period of symptom exacerbation has been reported (Kahn and Westenberg 1985; Kahn et al. 1987). About 30% to 50% of patients reported increased severity and frequency of panic attacks, as well as aggravation or induction of depressed mood during the initial 10 to 14 days of treatment. Continuation of treatment for 2 to 4 weeks eventually resulted in clinical improvement, when compared with pretreatment status (Kahn and Westenberg 1985; Kahn et al. 1987), both in terms of generalized anxiety and in the severity and frequency of the panic attacks. It is unlikely that this effect involves noradrenergic systems because it has also been reported using the selective 5-HT reuptake inhibitors fluvoxamine (Den Boer and Westenberg 1990b; Den Boer et al. 1987) and fluoxetine (Gorman et al. 1987). Thus, it appears that the initial anxiety to 5-HT agonist treatment in panic disorder is due to stimulation of 5-HT receptors. The biphasic effect of 5-HT agonists on anxiety might be explained by stimulation of hypersensitive 5-HT receptors, followed by a gradual,

Table 2-4. Serotonergic treatment studies in panic disorder

Author	Diagnosis (n)[a]	Drugs used	Dose (max) (mg/day)	Time (weeks)	Therapeutic effect[b]
Charney et al. (1987)	PD (74)	Trazodone Imipramine Alprazolam	250 (mean) 141 (mean) 3.1 (mean)	8	IMI = ALP > TRZ
Evans at al. (1986)	PD (25)	Zimelidine Imipramine Placebo	150 150	6	ZIM > IMI = PLA
Kahn et al. (1987)	PD (35) GAD (7)	5-Hydroxytryptophan Clomipramine Placebo	150 150	8	CMI = 5-HTP > PLA
Den Boer et al. (1987)	PD (50)	Clomipramine Fluvoxamine	150 100	8	CMI = FLU
Den Boer and Westenberg (1988)	PD (44)	Fluvoxamine Maprotiline	150 150	6	FLU > MAP

Cassano et al. (1988)	PD (59)	Clomipramine Imipramine	128 (mean) 144 (mean)	10	CMI = IMI[c]
Johnston et al. (1988)	A (108)	Clomipramine Placebo	83 (mean)	8	CMI > PLA
Sheehan et al. (1988)	PD (52)	Buspirone Imipramine Placebo	57 (mean) 292 (mean)	8	IMI ≥ BUSP ≥ PLA
Den Boer and Westenberg (1990b)	PD (60)	Fluvoxamine Ritanserin Placebo	150 20	8	FLU > RIT = PLA

Note.   All studies are parallel.
[a]PD = panic disorder; GAD = generalized anxiety disorder; A = agoraphobia.
[b]IMI = imipramine; ALP = alprazolam; TRZ = trazodone; ZIM = zimelidine; IMI = imipramine; PLA = placebo; CMI = clomipramine; 5-HTP = 5-hydroxytryptophan; FLU = fluvoxamine; MAP= maprotiline; BUSP = buspirone; RIT = ritanserin.
[c]Clomipramine had earlier effect than did imipramine.

compensatory downregulation of these receptors (Kahn and van Praag 1988).

Although the use of 5-HT reuptake inhibitors suggests a role for 5-HT in the treatment of panic anxiety, it does not provide information on which serotonergic system may be abnormal in panic disorder.

The recent availability of agents selective for a particular subset of 5-HT receptors for use in humans—such as the 5-HT$_{1A}$ partial agonists buspirone, gepirone, and ipsapirone; the selective 5-HT$_2$ antagonist ritanserin; and the selective 5-HT$_3$ antagonists GR 38242F and BRL 43694—may enable us to examine their efficacy in panic disorder and thus elucidate a possible role for these 5-HT receptors in the pathogenesis of this disorder. Only a very few studies with such agents have been conducted so far. One study comparing the antipanic effects of fluvoxamine with those of ritanserin and with placebo found that ritanserin was not effective in reducing panic symptoms (Den Boer and Westenberg 1990b). However, the dose of ritanserin used in this study (20 mg po) may have been too low to be efficacious. A study comparing the 5-HT$_{1A}$ partial agonist buspirone (60 mg po) with imipramine and placebo did not provide unambiguous data on the efficacy of buspirone. While imipramine was superior to placebo in reducing panic attacks and generalized anxiety symptoms, buspirone was neither more effective than placebo nor less effective than imipramine in reducing panic attacks (Sheehan et al. 1988).

In conclusion, the efficacy of 5-HT reuptake inhibitors in the treatment of panic attacks is well documented and replicated. However, the two studies using selective 5-HT antagonists provide less convincing results. Well-designed studies using adequate doses of selective 5-HT antagonists are required to test the role of these agents in the treatment of panic attacks.

Challenge studies.   The use of selective 5-HT agonists in panic disorder has provided some exciting and important new insights into the pathogenesis of this disorder (see Table 2–5). Several agents have been used, such as the 5-HT precursors tryptophan and 5-HTP, the 5-HT–releasing agent fenfluramine, and the direct 5-HT receptor agonist m-CPP. Although a number of studies have been conducted, most remain unreplicated.

m-Chlorophenylpiperazine is a direct 5-HT agonist that induces anxiety in humans. It binds strongly to 5-HT_{1A}, $5\text{-HT}_{1B/1D}$, $5\text{-HT}_{1C/2}$, and 5-HT_3 receptors (Hamik and Peroutka 1989; Hoyer 1988; Kilpatrick et al. 1987), exhibiting greatest affinity for the $5\text{-HT}_{1C/2}$ receptors (Hoyer 1988). Besides binding to 5-HT receptors, m-CPP also binds potently to α_2-adrenergic receptors (Hamik and Peroutka 1989; Smith and Suckow 1985). It binds weakly to α_1- and β-adrenergic receptors and very weakly to dopamine and muscarinic cholinergic receptors (Hamik and Peroutka 1989).

Given intravenously (0.1 mg/kg), m-CPP induced anxiety and

Table 2–5. Serotonergic challenge studies in panic disorder

Study	Challenge agent[a]	Diagnosis (n)[b]	Panic attacks Drug (%)	Panic attacks Placebo (%)	Hormonal effect[c]
Charney and Henninger (1986)	Tryptophan (7 g iv)	PD (23) NC (21)			P ↑ P ↑
Charney et al. (1987)	m-CPP/placebo (0.1 mg/kg iv)	PD (23) NC (19)	52 32	0 5	C ↑, P ↑ C↑, P ↑
Kahn et al. (1988a, 1988c)	m-CPP/placebo (0.25 mg/kg po)	PD (13) NC (15) MD (17)	45 5 10	0 0 0	C ↑ ↑ C = C =
Targum and Marshall (1989)	Fenfluramine/ placebo (60 mg po)	PD (9) MD (9) NC (9)	66 0 22	0 0 0	C ↑ ↑, P ↑ ↑ C =, P ↑ C =, P ↑
Den Boer and Westenberg (1990a)	5-HTP/placebo (60 mg iv)	PD (20) NC (20)	0 0	0 0	C ↑ ↑ C ↑ ↑
Klein et al. (1991)	m-CPP/caffeine/ placebo (m-CPP: 0.5 mg/kg po) (caffeine: 480 mg po)	PD (7)	70/70[d]	0	

[a]m-CPP = *m*-chlorophenylpiperazine; 5-HTP = 5-hydroxytryptophan.
[b]PD = panic disorder; NC = normal control; MD = major depression.
[c]P = prolactin; C = cortisol; ↑ = increase as compared with baseline or placebo; ↑↑ = augmented increase as compared with baseline or placebo; "=" indicates no change as compared with baseline or placebo.
[d]70% panic attacks on m-CPP and 70% panic attacks on caffeine.

panic in panic disorder patients and in normal control subjects (Charney et al. 1987). This effect appears to have been related to dose and route of administration, as we did not find anxiety induction in normal subjects using m-CPP in an oral dose of 0.5 mg/kg (Kahn et al. 1990). When an even lower oral dose (0.25 mg/kg) was used, m-CPP was found to increase anxiety and panic in panic disorder patients but not in normal control subjects (Kahn et al. 1988c). In another study, m-CPP (0.5 mg/kg po) induced panic attacks in five out of seven (70%) patients with panic disorder (versus none out of seven on placebo challenge) (Klein et al. 1991), whereas in normal subjects panic attacks either did not occur (Mueller et al. 1985; Murphy et al. 1989) or occurred in only 15% of the subjects (Kahn et al. 1990) at a dose of 0.25 mg/kg po m-CPP. These findings suggest that patients with panic disorder are hypersensitive to the anxiogenic effects of m-CPP, possibly because of increased postsynaptic 5-HT receptor sensitivity (Kahn and van Praag 1988).

Hormonal responses to m-CPP appear to corroborate these hypotheses. While a low oral dose of m-CPP (0.25 mg/kg) induced augmented cortisol release only in panic disorder patients (Kahn et al. 1988a), higher doses (e.g., 0.1 mg/kg m-CPP iv) resulted in increased cortisol levels in both patients and control subjects (Charney et al. 1987). Oral administration of 60 mg fenfluramine, a 5-HT agonist, appears to support the findings obtained with m-CPP. One study showed that fenfluramine induced anxiety and panic as well as augmented cortisol and prolactin release in (female) patients with panic disorder in contrast to normal control subjects and patients with major depression (Targum and Marshall 1989). Den Boer and Westenberg (1990a), using 5-HTP as a challenge agent, found similar cortisol release in both panic disorder patients and normal control subjects. However, because the majority of the normal subjects and 9 out of the 20 patients vomited during the test, the interpretation of these authors' results is problematic. The cortisol release is likely to have been stress-induced, rather than the result of 5-HTP– induced ACTH release. One study, using the 5-HT precursor tryptophan to challenge 5-HT receptors, found normal prolactin responses in patients with panic disorder (Charney and Heninger 1986).

These data can be explained by hypothesizing a presynaptic deficit in 5-HT in panic disorder. Tryptophan needs to be hydroxylated into 5-HTP, which is further decarboxylated into 5-HT. Any impairment in this process would lead to decreased presynaptic availability of 5-HT. Using the available data, it is most likely that an abnormality is present in the conversion process of tryptophan into 5-HTP. This is suggested by the failure of tryptophan to induce augmented prolactin responses in panic disorder patients. Indeed, the Charney and Heninger (1986) data suggest that prolactin release in response to tryptophan is lower, although not significantly, in panic disorder patients than it is in control subjects. When 5-HTP is administered, anxiety symptoms worsen, suggesting that 5-HTP is decarboxylated into 5-HT that then stimulates the postsynaptic receptors. This finding, in combination with the fenfluramine data (Targum and Marshall 1989), suggests that 5-HT release is normal in panic disorder. The augmented behavioral and hormonal response to m-CPP suggests that the postsynaptic $5\text{-HT}_{1C/2}$ or 5-HT_3 receptor is hypersensitive in panic disorder.

If indeed the conversion from tryptophan into 5-HTP is impaired in panic disorder, the availability of 5-HT in the synapse will be decreased and lead to decreased stimulation of the postsynaptic receptor, possibly resulting in adaptive increases in that receptor's sensitivity. Another adaptation mechanism would be to decrease the sensitivity of the 5-HT_{1A} autoreceptor, thereby lowering its inhibitory effect on 5-HT release. This hypothesis would explain the augmented responses to m-CPP and fenfluramine, and the normal to blunted response to tryptophan (Kahn and van Praag 1990).

Obsessive-Compulsive Disorder

Treatment studies. Evidence from challenge and treatment studies suggests that 5-HT is involved in the pathogenesis of OCD, although the nature of this involvement is unclear. Two studies measuring baseline CSF 5-HIAA in OCD patients yielded contradictory findings. Åsberg et al. (1982) found that a preponderance of females with OCD had low CSF 5-HIAA levels (as was found also in melancholic females). The average values, however, were no different from those of normal subjects. In contrast, Insel et al. (1985) found higher CSF 5-HIAA levels in OCD patients (males and females) compared with normal subjects. One possible explanation for this discrepancy in findings is the different sex distribution and the small sample size ($n = 8$) in Insel et al.'s study.

Clearer evidence for a 5-HT role in OCD comes from the increasing number of treatment studies reporting successful treatment of OCD with serotonergic agents (see Table 2–6). Several placebo-controlled studies involving clomipramine, a 5-HT reuptake inhibitor, demonstrated both antiobsessional and anticompulsive effects. In contrast, other tricyclic antidepressants with lesser or no effects on 5-HT reuptake, such as desmethylimipramine (Goodman et al. 1990b; Zohar and Insel 1987), nortriptyline (Thorén et al. 1980a), amitriptyline (Ananth et al. 1981), and imipramine (Foa et al. 1987; Volavka et al. 1985), have been found to be ineffective in treating OCD. Two studies noted a relationship between clinical improvement and clomipramine levels but no relationship to the levels of its noradrenergic metabolite (Insel et al. 1983; Stern et al. 1980). This would suggest that clomipramine's therapeutic effects are related to its 5-HT agonistic properties (see above) and not to its noradrenergic properties. In addition, improvement correlated well with reduction of CSF 5-HIAA concentration (Thorén et al. 1980b). Indeed, several placebo-controlled studies (see Table 2–4) have demonstrated the efficacy of the selective 5-HT reuptake inhibitor fluvoxamine (Goodman et al. 1989; Jenike et al. 1990b; Perse et al. 1987) in the treatment of OCD. However, the selective 5-HT reuptake inhibitor sertraline was ineffective in 19 OCD patients in a small placebo-controlled study (Jenike et al. 1990a). The failure to find a significant effect may have been due to the small number of subjects in each cell studied.

The overwhelming majority of studies suggest that 5-HT reuptake inhibitors are effective antiobsessional and anticompulsive agents when used as antidepressants in any psychiatric disorder. Moreover, only 5-HT reuptake inhibitors and not other antidepressants—such as the tricyclic antidepressants imipramine, desipramine, nortriptyline, and amitriptyline, and the monoamine oxidase inhibitor clorgyline (Table 2–4)—are effective in treating OCD. This strongly suggests that serotonergic systems may have a pathogenetic role in OCD.

Interestingly, but not surprisingly, 5-HT may not be the only neurotransmitter involved in the pathogenesis of OCD. Evidence suggests that in some OCD patients, in particular those with schizotypal personality disorder or those with tics, addition of a neuroleptic to the 5-HT reuptake inhibitors may improve treatment response (McDougle et al. 1990).

Challenge studies.   Challenge studies with m-CPP in OCD have provided important and intriguing findings (see Table 2–7). In one study (Zohar et al. 1987), m-CPP administration in OCD patients resulted in increased anxiety and obsessions as compared with normal control subjects, suggesting the presence of 5-HT receptor hypersensitivity. Yet cortisol response was blunted, and prolactin response was no different from that in normal subjects, indicating that 5-HT receptor hypersensitivity was not involved in 5-HT–mediated hormonal responses. Other investigators (Charney et al. 1988), however, failed to find exacerbation of OCD symptoms resulting from m-CPP challenge (0.1 mg/kg iv) or from tryptophan challenge (7 g iv). In contrast to the study by Zohar et al. (1987), Charney et al. (1988) found blunted prolactin response in female OCD patients as compared with normal control subjects, but they found no differences in cortisol response between the two groups. Although the present data indicate a role for 5-HT in OCD, the exact nature of its role is far from clear.

On rechallenge with m-CPP following 3.5 months of clomipramine treatment, the induction of anxiety and obsessions was absent (Zohar et al. 1988), suggesting that downregulation of 5-HT receptors had occurred. Similarly, 12-week treatment with 80 mg/day of the selective 5-HT reuptake inhibitor fluoxetine (Hollander et al. 1989b) reduced the behavioral effects of m-CPP (0.5 mg/kg po) observed in these patients during their premedication state. Another study confirmed that during treatment with clomipramine or fluoxetine, m-CPP induced no behavioral effects (Pigott et al. 1990).

These findings have been explained as follows. The m-CPP–induced aggravation of obsessive symptoms suggests that in-

Table 2–6. Serotonergic treatment studies in obsessive-compulsive disorder

Author	Drug	Compared with	Number of patients	Number of weeks	Maximum dose (mg/day)	Effect[a]
Thorén et al. (1980a)	Clomipramine Nortriptyline	Placebo	35	5	150 150	CMI > NOR = PLA
Marks et al. (1980)	Clomipramine	Placebo	40	4	225	CMI > PLA
Montgomery (1980)	Clomipramine	Placebo	14	4[b]	75	CMI > PLA
Ananth et al. (1981)	Clomipramine	Amitriptyline	20	4	300/300	CMI > AMI
Insel et al. (1983)	Clomipramine Clorgyline	Placebo	13	4 + 6[b]	300 30	CMI > CLO = PLA
Insel et al. (1985)	Zimelidine Desipramine Clomipramine	Placebo	13	5[b]	300 300 300	CMI > DMI = ZIM = PLA
Mavissakalian et al. (1985)	Clomipramine	Placebo	15	12	229[c]	CMI > PLA
Volavka et al. (1985)	Clomipramine	Imipramine	23	12	300/300	CMI > IMI

Foa et al. (1987)	Imipramine	Placebo	37	6	233[c]	IMI = PLA
Perse et al. (1987)	Fluvoxamine	Placebo	16	20[b]	300	FLU > PLA
Zohar and Insel (1987)	Clomipramine	Desipramine	10	6	300	CMI > DMI
Goodman et al. (1989)	Fluvoxamine	Placebo	42	6	300	FLU > PLA
Goodman et al. (1990b)	Fluvoxamine	Desipramine	40	8	300/300	FLU > DMI
Jenike et al. (1990b)	Fluvoxamine	Placebo	38	10	300	FLU > PLA
Jenike et al. (1990a)	Sertraline	Placebo	19	10	200	SER = PLA

Note. All comparative studies are parallel unless stated differently.
[a]CMI = clomipramine; NOR = nortriptyline; PLA = placebo; AMI = amitriptyline; CLO = clorgyline; DMI = desipramine; ZIM = zimelidine; IMI = imipramine; FLU = fluvoxamine; SER = sertraline.
[b]Crossover design.
[c]Mean mg/day.

Table 2–7. Serotonergic challenge studies in obsessive-compulsive disorder

Authors	Drug (dose)[a]	Diagnosis (n)[b]	Hormonal effects[c]	Behavioral effects[d]	Other effects[e]
Zohar et al. (1987)	m-CPP/placebo (0.5 mg/kg po)	OCD (15), NC (20)	C: OCD < NC, P: OCD = NC	OCD: anx ↑, obsess ↑,	T: OCD < NC
Charney et al. (1988)	m-CPP/placebo (0.1 mg/kg iv)	OCD (21), NC (21)	P: OCD_F < NC_F, C: OCD = NC	OCD = NC	
Charney et al. (1988)	Tryptophan/placebo (7 g iv)	OCD (21), NC (21)	P: OCD = NC, C: OCD = NC	OCD = NC	
Zohar et al. (1988)	m-CPP (0.5 mg/kg po)	OCD −CMI (9), OCD +CMI (9)	P: −CMI = +CMI, C: −CMI = +CMI	− CMI: anx ↑, obsess ↑, + CMI: anx =, obsess =	T: +CMI < −CMI
Hollander et al. (1988, 1989a)	m-CPP/placebo (0.5 mg/kg po)	OCD (20), NC (10)	P: OCD < NC, C: OCD < NC	OCD: obsess ↑	
Hollander et al. (1989b)	m-CPP (0.5 mg/kg po)	OCD −FLX (6), OCD +FLX (6)	P: −FLX < +FLX	− FLX: obsess ↑, + FLX: obsess =	
Pigott et al. (1990)	m-CPP (0.5 mg/kg po)	OCD +CMI (6), OCD +FLX (11)	P: CMI = FLX, C: CMI > FLX	+ FLX: obsess =, + CMI: obsess =	

[a]m-CPP = m-chlorophenylpiperazine.
[b]OCD = obsessive-compulsive disorder; NC = normal control; −CMI = after clomipramine treatment; +CMI = prior to clomipramine treatment; −FLX = after fluoxetine treatment; +FLX = prior to fluoxetine treatment.
[c]C = cortisol; P = prolactin; subscript F indicates female subjects.
[d]↑/↓, = increase/decrease; "=" indicates no change. "obsess" indicates obsessions and "anx" indicates anxiety.
[e]T = temperature.

creased 5-HT function is a pathogenetic mechanism in OCD. Chronic treatment with a 5-HT agonist, such as clomipramine or fluvoxamine, reduces the sensitivity of postsynaptic 5-HT receptors (possibly as an adaptive mechanism to increased availability of 5-HT at the receptor site). Rechallenge with a 5-HT agonist, then, fails to induce an exacerbation of OCD symptoms because receptor sensitivity has been normalized as a result of the antidepressant treatment. However, this hypothesis was challenged in a recent study in which 10 OCD patients who were treated with clomipramine for from 2.5 up to 24 months received an additional 4 mg/day of metergoline or placebo in a crossover design for 4 days. Patients experienced increased anxiety and obsessive and compulsive symptoms when metergoline was added (Benkelfat et al. 1989). Although these results strongly suggest that clomipramine is effective through its effect on serotonergic systems, these findings dispute the hypothesis that clomipramine (and other 5-HT reuptake inhibitors) is effective by downregulation of 5-HT receptor sensitivity (i.e., decreasing 5-HT activity). Indeed, a more likely explanation of these findings is that clomipramine is effective in OCD because it increases 5-HT function. This conclusion, however, is difficult to reconcile with the finding that OCD symptoms worsen after challenge with a 5-HT agonist (i.e., m-CPP). In summary, a hypothesis explaining these disparate findings is still lacking.

Generalized Anxiety Disorder

Evidence that 5-HT function may be involved in GAD has been obtained from several treatment studies using 5-HT agents. Two new drugs, buspirone and ritanserin, both having pronounced effects on serotonergic systems, have been shown to be effective in treating GAD. In most investigations, buspirone has proven to be as anxiolytic as the benzodiazepines (Cohn and Wilcox 1986; Cohn et al. 1986; Goldberg and Finnerty 1979, 1982; Olajide and Lader 1987; Rickels et al. 1982; Ross and Matas 1987; Wheatley 1982).

Buspirone appears to exert its influence through the 5-HT_{1A} receptor, for which it has a high affinity. Although it also binds to D_2 sites, its affinity at these sites is 16 times weaker (Peroutka

1985) and so is probably less significant clinically. Buspirone has been noted to have both agonistic and antagonistic effects on 5-HT_{1A} receptors. Its net effect, however, is probably to decrease 5-HT function, because administration of buspirone decreases raphe cell activity (Van der Maelen and Wildeman 1984).

Preliminary results involving the selective 5-HT_2 antagonist ritanserin showed that it is also effective in treating GAD (Leysen et al. 1985). Administered for 2 weeks (10 mg/day) in a placebo-controlled study ($N = 83$), ritanserin was found to be more effective than placebo, and as effective as lorazepam, in a group of GAD patients (Ceulemans et al. 1985b). Another study ($N = 191$) comparing ritanserin (10 mg/day) with placebo and diazepam (10 mg/day) found ritanserin, after 3 weeks of treatment, to be more effective than diazepam or placebo (Ceulemans et al. 1985a). Its therapeutic effect, however, may be dose related, because a lower dose (5 mg/day) of ritanserin appeared to be ineffective (Ceulemans et al. 1985b).

Anxiety in Depressive Disorders

A relationship between 5-HT and anxiety in major depression is suggested by the findings that anxiety is often a prominent component of affective disorders and that 5-HT has been implicated in the pathogenesis of depression. Only a few studies, however, have investigated this relationship directly. Both Banki (1977) and Rydin et al. (1982) found an inverse correlation between CSF 5-HIAA and anxiety in depressed patients. Redmond et al. (1986) also found such a correlation, though it was less pronounced than the relationship between anxiety and 3-methoxy-4-hydroxy-phenylglycol (MHPG, the main metabolite of norepinephrine). Clearly, more studies are needed to investigate the role of serotonergic and other neurotransmitter systems in depressive/anxiety states.

Conclusion: Serotonin and Human Anxiety

Studies examining the role of 5-HT in human anxiety suggest that 5-HT reuptake inhibitors are effective in the treatment of panic disorder and OCD and that 5-HT_{1A} partial agonists and 5-HT_2 antagonists are effective in the treatment of GAD. Moreover, a single dose of the direct 5-HT agonist m-CPP induces anxiety in human subjects, an effect that is augmented in panic disorder and OCD patients. Fenfluramine, another 5-HT agonist, also elicits augmented anxiety in patients with panic disorder. Hypersensitivity of (some) 5-HT receptors in panic disorder and OCD has been hypothesized to explain these findings. 5-HT reuptake inhibitors may be effective by downregulation of these hypersensitive 5-HT receptors.

CONCLUSIONS

In this chapter we have reviewed the animal and human findings concerning the relationship between 5-HT function and anxiety. It may be concluded that in animals and humans, increasing 5-HT function is anxiogenic. In animals, and possibly in humans, decreasing 5-HT function is anxiolytic. The findings reviewed above raise several questions.

First, does the evidence of 5-HT dysfunction found in panic disorder, OCD, and possibly GAD suggest that each diagnosis is related to different 5-HT abnormalities, or that these disorders share a common 5-HT abnormality related to a psychopathological dimension such as anxiety (van Praag et al. 1990)? There is evidence for both alternatives. Although m-CPP induces anxiety in both panic disorder and OCD patients, and 5-HT reuptake inhibitors are effective in both disorders, in OCD patients m-CPP induces blunted hormone responses (Hollander et al. 1989a; Zohar et al. 1988), while in panic disorder patients hormone release is augmented (Kahn et al. 1988a; Targum and Marshall 1989). 5-HT$_{1A}$ partial agonists and 5-HT$_2$ antagonists may be effective in the treatment of GAD but ineffective in the treatment of panic disorder (Den Boer and Westenberg 1990b; Sheehan et al. 1988).

Second, although the data reviewed suggest that 5-HT dysfunction is present in panic disorder, OCD, and GAD patients, these data do not provide information on which 5-HT receptor(s) is involved in the pathogenesis of these disorders. For instance, 5-HT$_{1A}$ partial agonists and 5-HT$_2$ antagonists appear to be effective anxiolytics in patients with GAD (see Table 2–5) but may not be effective antipanic agents. (However, as mentioned above, the doses used may have been too low to treat panic anxiety vs. generalized anxiety.) Does this suggest that $5\text{-}HT_{1A}$ and $5\text{-}HT_2$ receptor abnormalities are present in GAD but not in panic disorder? Will $5\text{-}HT_3$ receptor antagonists be effective antipanic agents and/or antiobsessional agents? Addressing these questions is now possible because agents selective for the $5\text{-}HT_{1A}$, $5\text{-}HT_2$, and $5\text{-}HT_3$ receptors have become available.

Third, 5-HT dysfunction has been associated with forms of psychopathology other than anxiety, including depressive disorders (van Praag and Korf 1971), suicidal behavior (for review, see van Praag 1986), and outwardly directed aggression (for review, see Cocarro 1989). Again, the question arises as to whether each disorder is independently related to particular disturbances of the central 5-HT system, or whether a particular 5-HT disturbance is linked to a particular psychopathological trait common to all the disorders, such as anxiety.

Finally, 5-HT dysfunction is not the only abnormality hypothesized to be involved in anxiety. Increased noradrenergic function has been proposed as a pathogenic factor in panic attacks (Charney and Redmond 1983; Redmond and Huang 1979), while the benzodiazepine–gamma-aminobutyric acid (GABA) complex has been suggested as playing a role in anxiety (Paul et al. 1981). As indicated earlier, there is increasing evidence that abnormal dopaminergic function may contribute to OCD (Goodman et al. 1990a). How can one reconcile the role of 5-HT in the pathogenesis of anxiety with the evidence of noradrenergic, GABAergic, and possibly dopaminergic involvement as well? Several possible explanations may be considered. For example, certain anxiety states may be related to a predominant dysfunction of one neurotransmitter system, while other anxiety states may be related to disturbances in another neurotransmitter system. Alternatively, because serotonergic and noradrenergic (Descarries and Leger 1978; Leger et al. 1979; Pickel et al. 1978), serotonergic and GABAergic (Belin et al. 1983; Nanopoulos et al. 1982), and serotonergic and dopaminergic (see Goodman et al. 1990a) systems have extensive connecting pathways, a disturbance in one may cause secondary or complementary effects in the other. Indeed, functionally, 5-HT neurons have clear-cut effects on these other neurotransmitter systems and vice versa.

In conclusion, although there is increasing evidence of a role for 5-HT in anxiety, these findings have raised several important questions. With the advent of new compounds selective for each subset of 5-HT receptors, some of these questions may be answered in the near future, leading, hopefully, to a more specific treatment for anxiety. However, even at this time, research into the role of 5-HT in anxiety has produced important and tangible results for the clinical care of the anxious patient.

REFERENCES

Ananth J, Pecknold JC, van der Steen N: Double-blind comparative study of clomipramine and amitriptyline in obsessive-compulsive neurosis. Progress in Neuro-Psychopharmacology 5:257–264, 1981

Åsberg M, Thorén P, Bertilsson L: Clomipramine treatment of obsessive-compulsive disorder: biochemical and clinical aspects. Psychopharmacol Bull 18:13–21, 1982

Aulakh CS, Wozniak KM, Haas M, et al: Food intake, neuroendocrine and temperature effects of 8-OHDPAT in the rat. Eur J Pharmacol 146:235–259, 1988

Azmitia EC, Segal M: An autoradiographic analysis of the differential ascending projections of the dorsal and median raphe nuclei in the rat. J Comp Neurol 179:641–667, 1978

Banki CM: Correlation of anxiety and related symptoms with cerebrospinal fluid 5-hydroxyindoleacetic acid in depressed women. J Neural Transm 41:135–143, 1977

Barofski AL, Grier HC, Pradkan TK: Evidence for regulation of water intake by median raphe 5-HT neurons. Physiol Behav 24:951–955, 1980

Belin MF, Nanopoulos D, Didier M, et al: Immunohistochemical evidence for the presence of gamma-aminobutyric acid and serotonin in one nerve cell: a study on the raphe nuclei of the rat using antibodies to glutamate decarboxylase and serotonin. Brain Res 275:329–339, 1983

Benjamin D, Harbans L, Meyerson LR: The effects of 5-HT$_{1B}$ characterizing agents in the mouse elevated plus-maze. Life Sci 47:195–203, 1990

Benkelfat C, Murphy DL, Zohar J, et al: Clomipramine in obsessive-compulsive disorder. Arch Gen Psychiatry 46:23–28, 1989

Blakely TA, Parker LF: The effects of parachlorophenylalanine on experimentally induced conflict behavior. Pharmacol Biochem Behav 1:609–613, 1973

Blundell JE: Serotonin and appetite. Neuropharmacology 23(12B):1537–1551, 1984

Briley M, Chopin P, Moret C: Effect of serotonergic lesion on "anxious" behaviour measured in the elevated plus-maze test in the rat. Psychopharmacology (Berlin) 101:187–189, 1990

Cassano GB, Petracca A, Perugi G, et al: Clomipramine for panic disorder, I: the first 10 weeks of a long-term comparison with imipramine. J Affective Disord 14:123–127, 1988

Ceulemans DLS, Hoppenbrouwers ML, Gelders YG, et al: The effect of benzodiazepine withdrawal on the therapeutic efficacy of a serotonin antagonist in anxiety disorders. Paper presented at the IVth World Congress of Biological Psychiatry, Philidephia, PA, September 1985a

Ceulemans DLS, Hoppenbrouwers ML, Gelders YG, et al: The influence of ritanserin, a serotonin antagonist, in anxiety disorders: a double-blind placebo-controlled study versus lorazepam. Pharmacopsychiatry 18:303–305, 1985b

Charney DS, Heninger GR: Serotonergic function in panic disorders. Arch Gen Psychiatry 43:1059–1065, 1986

Charney DS, Redmond DE Jr: Neurobiological mechanisms in human anxiety: evidence supporting central noradrenergic hyperactivity. Neuropharmacology 22:1531–1536, 1983

Charney DS, Woods SW, Goodman WK, et al: Serotonin function in anxiety, II: effects of the serotonin agonist mCPP in panic disorder patients and healthy subjects. Psychopharmacology (Berlin) 92:14–24, 1987

Charney DS, Goodman WK, Price LH, et al: Serotonin function in obsessive-compulsive disorder: a comparison of the effects of tryptophan and m-chlorophenylpiperazine in patients and healthy subjects. Arch Gen Psychiatry 45:177–185, 1988

Clarke A, File SE: Selective neurotoxin lesions of the lateral septum: changes in social and aggressive behaviours. Pharmacol Biochem Behav 17:623–628, 1982

Coccaro EF: Central serotonin and impulsive aggression. Br J Psychiatry 155:52–62, 1989

Cohn JB, Wilcox C: Low-sedation potential of buspirone compared with alprazolam and lorazepam in the treatment of anxious patients: a double-blind study. J Clin Psychiatry 47:409–412, 1986

Cohn JB, Bowden CL, Fisher JG, et al: Double-blind comparison of buspirone and clorazepate in anxious outpatients. Am J Med 80(3B):10–16, 1986

Colpaert FC, Meert TF, Niemegeers CJE, et al: Behavioral and 5-HT antagonist effects of ritanserin: a pure and selective antagonist of LSD discrimination in the rat. Psychopharmacology (Berlin) 86:45–54, 1985

Commissaris RL, Rech RH: Interactions of metergoline with diazepam, quipazine and hallucinogenic drugs on a conflict behavior in the rat. Psychopharmacology (Berlin) 76:282, 1982

Commissaris RL, Lyness WH, Rech RH: The effects of d-lysergic acid diethylamide (LSD), 2,5-dimethoxy-4-methylamphetamine (DOM), pentobarbital and methaqualone on punished responding in control and 5,7-dihydroxytryptamine-treated rats. Pharmacol Biochem Behav 14:617–623, 1981

Conn PJ, Sanders-Bush E, Hoffman BJ, et al: A unique serotonin receptor in choroid plexus is linked to phosphatidylinositol turnover. Proc Natl Acad Sci U S A 83:4086–4088, 1986

Cook L, Sepinwall J: Behavioral analysis of the effects and mechanism of action of benzodiazepines, in Mechanism of Action of Benzodiazepines. Edited by Costa E, Greengard P. New York, Raven, 1975, pp 1–28

Costall B, Domeney AM, Gerrard PA, et al: Effects of the 5-HT receptor antagonist GR 38032F, ICS205-930 and BRL43694 in tests for anxiolytic activity. Br J Pharmacol 90:195P, 1987

Crawley J, Goodwin FK: Preliminary report of a simple animal behavior model for the anxiolytic effects of benzodiazepines. Pharmacol Biochem Behav 13:167–170, 1980

Critchley MAE, Handley SL: Effects in the X-maze anxiety model of agents acting at the 5-HT$_1$ and 5-HT$_2$ receptors. Psychopharmacology (Berlin) 93:502–506, 1987

Den Boer JA, Westenberg HGM: Effect of a serotonin and noradrenaline uptake inhibitor in panic disorder: a double-blind comparative study with fluvoxamine and maprotiline. Int Clin Psychopharmacol 3:59–74, 1988

Den Boer JA, Westenberg HGM: Behavioral, neuroendocrine and biochemical effects of 5-hydroxytryptophan administration in panic disorder. Psychiatry Res 31:267–278, 1990a

Den Boer JA, Westenberg HGM: Serotonin function in panic disorder: a double-blind placebo-controlled study with fluvoxamine and ritanserin. Psychopharmacology (Berlin) 102:85–94, 1990b

Den Boer JA, Westenberg HGM, Kamerbeek WDJ, et al: Effect of serotonin uptake inhibitors in anxiety disorders; a double-blind comparison of clomipramine and fluvoxamine. Int Clin Psychopharmacol 2:21–32, 1987

Descarries L, Leger L: Serotonin nerve terminals in the locus coeruleus of the adult rat, in Interactions Between Putative Neurotransmitters in the Brain. Edited by Garattini S, Pujol JF, Samanin R. New York, Raven, 1978, pp 355–367

Ellison GD: Animal models of psychopathology: the low-norepineph-rine and low-serotonin rat. Am Psychol 32:1036–1045, 1977

Engel JA, Hjorth S, Svensson K, et al: Anticonflict effect of the putative serotonin receptor agonist 8-hydroxy-2-(di-n-propylamino)tetralin (8-OH-DPAT). Eur J Pharmacol 105:365–368, 1984

Estes WK, Skinner BF: Some quantitative properties of anxiety. Journal of Experimental Psychology 29:390–400, 1941

Evans L, Moore G: The treatment of phobic anxiety by zimelidine. Acta Psychiatr Scand Suppl 63:290:342–345, 1981

Evans L, Kenardy J, Schneider P, et al: Effect of a selective serotonin uptake inhibitor in agoraphobia with panic attacks. Acta Psychiatr Scand 73:49–53, 1986

Fargin A, Raymond JR, Lohse MJ, et al: The genomic clone G-21 which resembles a β-adrenergic receptor sequence encodes the 5-HT$_{1a}$ receptor. Nature 335:358–360, 1988

File SE: Animal models for predicting clinical efficacy of anxiolytic drugs: social behaviour. Neuropsychobiology 13:55–62, 1985

File SE, Hyde JR: The effects of p-chlorophenylalanine and ethanolam-ine-O-sulphate in an animal test of anxiety. J Pharm Pharmacol 29:735–738, 1977

File SE, Hyde JRG, Macleod NK: 5,7-Dihydroxytryptamine lesions of dorsal and median raphe nuclei and performance in the social inter-action test of anxiety and in a home-cage aggression test. J Affective Disord 1:115–122, 1979

Foa EB, Steketee G, Kozak MJ, et al: Effects of imipramine on depression and obsessive-compulsive symptoms. Psychiatry Res 21:123–136, 1987

Gardner CR: in Neuropharmacology of Serotonin. Edited by Green RA. New York, Oxford University Press, 1985, pp 281–325

Gardner CR: Recent developments in 5-HT-related pharmacology of animal models of anxiety. Pharmacol Biochem Behav 24:1479–1485, 1986

Geller I, Blum K: The effects of 5-HTP on para-chlorophenylalanine (p-CPA) attenuation of "conflict" behavior. Eur J Pharmacol 9:319–324, 1970

Geller I, Seifter J: The effects of meprobamate, d-amphetamine and pro-mazine on experimentally-induced conflict in the rat. Psychopharma-cologica 1:482–492, 1960

Geller I, Hartmann RJ, Croy DJ, et al: Attenuation of conflict behavior with cinanserin, a serotonin antagonist: reversal of the effect with 5-hydroxytryptophan and -methyltryptamine. Res Commun Chem Pathol Pharmacol 7:165–175, 1974

Gilbert F, Dourish CT, Brazell C, et al: Relationship of increased food intake and plasma ACTH levels to 5-HT1a receptor activation in rats. Neuroendocrinology 13:471–478, 1988

Goldberg HL, Finnerty RJ: The comparative efficacy of buspirone and diazepam in the treatment of anxiety. Am J Psychiatry 136:1184–1187, 1979

Goldberg HL, Finnerty RJ: Comparison of buspirone in two separate studies. J Clin Psychiatry 43:87–92, 1982

Goodman WK, Price LH, Rasmussen SA, et al: Efficacy of fluvoxamine in obsessive-compulsive disorder. Arch Gen Psychiatry 46:36–44, 1989

Goodman WK, McDougle CJ, Price LH, et al: Beyond the serotonin hypothesis: a role for dopamine in some forms of obsessive-compulsive disorder? J Clin Psychiatry 51 (no 8, suppl):36–43, 1990a

Goodman WK, Price LH, Delgado PL, et al: Specificity of serotonin reuptake inhibitors in the treatment of obsessive-compulsive disorder. Arch Gen Psychiatry 47:577–585, 1990b

Gorman JM, Liebowitz MR, Fyer AJ, et al: An open trial of fluoxetine in the treatment of panic attacks. J Clin Psychopharmacol 7:329–332, 1987

Graeff FG: Tryptamine antagonists and punished behavior. J Pharmacol Exp Ther 189:344–350, 1974

Graeff FG, Schoenfeld RI: Tryptaminergic mechanisms in punished and nonpunished behavior. J Pharmacol Exp Ther 173:277–283, 1970

Hamik A, Peroutka SJ: 1-m-Chlorophenyl piperazine (MCPP) interactions with neurotransmitter receptors in the human brain. Biol Psychiatry 25:569–575, 1989

Heuring RE, Peroutka SJ: Characterization of a novel 3H-5-hydroxytryptamine binding site subtype in bovine brain membranes. J Neurosci 7:894–903, 1987

Hollander E, Fay M, Cohen B, et al: Serotonergic and noradrenergic sensitivity in obsessive-compulsive disorder: behavioral findings. Am J Psychiatry 145:1015–1018, 1988

Hollander E, DeCaria C, Cooper T, et al: Neuroendocrine sensitivity in obsessive-compulsive disorder. Biol Psychiatry 25(suppl):5A-9A, 1989a

Hollander E, DeCaria C, Fay M, et al: Repeat MCPP challenge during fluoxetine treatment in obsessive-compulsive disorder: behavioral and neuroendocrine responses. Biol Psychiatry 25(suppl):5A–9A, 1989b

Hoyer D: Functional correlates of serotonin 5-HT1 recognition sites. Journal Receptor Research 8:59–81, 1988

Hoyer D, Pazos A, Probst A, et al: Serotonin receptors in the human brain, I: characterization and autoradiographic localization of 5-HT$_{1A}$ recognition sites: apparent absence of 5-HT$_{1B}$ recognition sites. Brain Res 376:85–96, 1986a

Hoyer D, Pazos A, Probst A, et al: Serotonin receptors in the human brain, II: characterization and autoradiographic localization of 5-HT$_{1C}$ and 5-HT$_2$ recognition sites. Brain Res 376:97–107, 1986b

Insel TR, Murphy DL, Cohen RM, et al: Obsessive-compulsive disorder: a double-blind trial of clomipramine and clorgyline. Arch Gen Psychiatry 40:605–612, 1983

Insel TR, Mueller EA, Alterman I, et al: Obsessive-compulsive disorder and serotonin: is there a connection? Biol Psychiatry 20:1174–1188, 1985

Jenike MA, Baer L, Summergrad P, et al: Sertraline in obsessive-compulsive disorder: a double-blind comparison with placebo. Am J Psychiatry 147:928–932, 1990a

Jenike MA, Hyman S, Baer L, et al: A controlled trial of fluvoxamine in obsessive-compulsive disorder: implications for a serotonergic theory. Am J Psychiatry 147:1209–1215, 1990b

Johnston DG, Troyer IE, Whitsett SF: Clomipramine treatment of agoraphobic women. Arch Gen Psychiatry 45:453–459, 1988

Jones BJ, Oakley NR, Tyers MB: The anxiolytic activity of GR38032F, a 5-HT$_3$ antagonist, in the rat and cynomolgus monkey (abstract). Br J Pharmacol 90:88P, 1987

Julius D, MacDermot AB, Axel R, et al: Molecular characterization of a functional cDNA encoding the serotonin 1c receptor. Science 241:558–564, 1988

Kahn RS, van Praag HM: A serotonin hypothesis of panic disorder. Human Psychopharmacology 3:285–288, 1988

Kahn RS, van Praag HM: Panic disorder: a pre-synaptic serotonin defect? Psychiatry Res 31:209–210, 1990

Kahn RS, Westenberg HGM: l-5-Hydroxytryptophan in the treatment of anxiety disorders. J Affective Disord 8:197–200, 1985

Kahn RS, Westenberg HGM, Verhoeven WMA, et al: Effect of a serotonin precursor and uptake inhibitor in anxiety disorders: a double-blind comparison of 5-hydroxytryptophan, clomipramine and placebo. Int Clin Psychopharmacol 2:33–45, 1987

Kahn RS, Asnis GM, Wetzler S, et al: Neuroendocrine evidence for serotonin receptor hypersensitivity in patients with panic disorder. Psychopharmacology (Berlin) 96:360–364, 1988a

Kahn RS, van Praag HM, Wetzler S, et al: Serotonin and anxiety revisited. Biol Psychiatry 23:189–208, 1988b

Kahn RS, Wetzler S, van Praag HM, et al: Behavioral indications of serotonergic supersensitivity in patients with panic disorder. Psychiatry Res 25:101–104, 1988c

Kahn RS, Wetzler S, Asnis GM, et al: The effects of m-chlorophenyl-piperazine in normal subjects: a dose-response study. Psychopharmacology (Berlin) 100:339–344, 1990

Kennett GA, Whitton P, Shah K, et al: Anxiogenic-like effects of mCPP and TFMPP in animal models are opposed by 5-HT$_{1c}$ receptor antagonists. Eur J Pharmacol 164:445–454, 1989

Kilpatrick GJ, Jones BJ, Tyers MB: Identification and distribution of 5-HT$_3$ receptors in rat brain using radioligand binding. Nature 330:746–748, 1987

Kilts CD, Commissaris RL, Rech RH: Comparison of anti-conflict drug effects in three experimental animal models of anxiety. Psychopharmacology (Berlin) 74:290–296, 1981

Kilts CD, Commissaris RL, Cordon JJ, et al: Lack of central 5-hydroxy-tryptamine influence on the anticonflict activity of diazepam. Psychopharmacology (Berlin) 78:156–164, 1982

Klein E, Zohar J, Geraci MF, et al: Anxiogenic effects on m-CPP in patients with panic disorder: comparison to caffeine's anxiogenic effects. Biol Psychiatry 30:973–989, 1991

Kokzacks S, Holmberg G, Wedin L: A pilot study of the effect of the 5-HT-uptake inhibitor, zimelidine, on phobic anxiety. Acta Psychiatr Scand Suppl 290:328–341, 1981

Krulich L, McCann SM, Mayfield MA: On the mode of the prolactin release–inhibiting action of the serotonin receptor blockers metergoline, methysergide, and cyproheptadine. Endocrinology 108:1115–1124, 1981

Leger L, Wiklund L, Descarries L, et al: Description of an indolaminergic cell component in the cat locus coeruleus: a fluorescence histochemical and radioautographic study. Brain Res 168:43–56, 1979

Leone CML, de Aguiar JC, Graeff FG: Role of 5-hydroxytryptamine in amphetamine effects on unpunished behavior. Psychopharmacology (Berlin) 80:78–82, 1983

Leysen JE, Gommeren W, van Gompel P: Receptor binding properties in vitro and in vivo of ritanserin: a very potent and long-acting 5-HT$_2$ antagonist. Mol Pharmacol 27:600–611, 1985

Liebowitz MR: Imipramine in the treatment of panic disorder and its complications. Psychiatr Clin North Am 8:37–47, 1985

Lippa AS, Nash PA, Greenblatt EN: Preclinical neuropsycho- pharmacological testing procedures for anxiolytic drugs, in Industrial Pharmacology. Edited by Fielding S, Lal H. New York, Futura, 1979, pp 3–41

Marks IM, Stern RS, Mawson D, et al: Clomipramine and exposure for obsessive-compulsive rituals. Br J Psychiatry 136:1–25, 1980

Mavissakalian M: Trazodone in the treatment of panic agoraphobia, in New Research Program and Abstracts, 139th annual meeting of the American Psychiatric Association, Washington, DC, May 1986

Mavissakalian M, Turner S, Michelson L, et al: Tricyclic antidepressants in obsessive-compulsive disorder: antiobsessional or antidepressant agents? II. Am J Psychiatry 142:572–576, 1985

McDougle CJ, Goodman WK, Price LH, et al: Neuroleptic addition in fluvoxamine-refractory obsessive-compulsive disorder. Am J Psychiatry 147:652–654, 1990

Montgomery KC: The relation between fear induced by novel stimulation and exploratory behavior. Journal of Comparative and Physiological Psychology 48:254–260, 1955

Montgomery SA: Clomipramine in obsessional neurosis: a placebo controlled trial. Pharmacological Medicine 1:189–192, 1980

Mueller EA, Sunderland T, Murphy DL: Neuroendocrine effects of m-CPP, a serotonin agonist, in humans. J Clin Endocrinol Metab 61:1179–1184, 1985

Murphy DL, Mueller EA, Hill JL, et al: Comparative anxiogenic, neuroendocrine, and other physiologic effects of m-chlorophenylpiperazine given intravenously or orally to healthy volunteers. Psychopharmacology (Berlin) 98:275–282, 1989

Nanopoulos D, Belin MF, Maitre M, et al: Immunocytochemical evidence for the existence of GABAergic neurons in the nucleus raphe dorsalis: possible existence of neurons containing serotonin and GABA. Brain Res 232:375–389, 1982

Olajide D, Lader M: A comparison of buspirone, diazepam and placebo in patients with chronic anxiety states. J Clin Psychopharmacol 7:148–152, 1987

Papp M: Similar effects of diazepam and the 5-HT$_3$ receptor antagonist ICS205930 on place aversion conditioning. Eur J Pharmacol 151:321–324, 1988

Paul SM, Marangos PJ, Skolnick P: The benzodiazepine-GABA-chloride ionophore receptor complex: common site of minor tranquilizer action. Biol Psychiatry 16:213–229, 1981

Pellow S, Johnston AL, File SE: Selective agonists and antagonists for 5-hydroxytryptamine receptor subtypes, and interactions with yohimbine and FG 7142 using the elevated plus-maze test in the rat. J Pharm Pharmacol 39:917–928, 1987

Peroutka SJ: Selective interaction of novel anxiolytics with 5-hydroxytryptamine $_{1a}$ receptors. Biol Psychiatry 20:971–979, 1985

Perse TL, Greist JH, Jefferson JW, et al: Fluvoxamine treatment of obsessive-compulsive disorder. Am J Psychiatry 144:1543–1548, 1987

Petersen EN, Lassen JB: A water lick conflict paradigm using drug experienced rats. Psychopharmacology (Berlin) 75:236–239, 1981

Pickel VM, Tong HJ, Reis DJ: Immunocytochemical evidence for serotonergic innervation of noradrenergic neurons in nucleus locus coeruleus, in Interactions Between Putative Neurotransmitters in the Brain. Edited by Garattini S, Pujol JF, Samanin R. New York, Raven, 1978, pp 369–382

Pigott TA, Yoney TH, L'Heureux F, et al: Serotonergic responsivity to m-CPP in OCD patients during clomipramine and fluoxetine treatment. Biol Psychiatry 27:41A–179A, 1990

Piper D, Upton N, Thomas D, et al: The effects of the 5-HT$_3$ receptor antagonists BRL 43694 and GR 38042F in animal behavioral models of anxiety. Br J Pharmacol 91:314P, 1987

Pritchett DB, Bach AW, Wozny M, et al: Structure and functional expression of cloned rat serotonin 5-HT$_2$ receptor. EMBO J 7:4135–4140, 1988

Redmond DE Jr, Huang YH: Current concepts, II: new evidence for a locus coeruleus-norepinephrine connection with anxiety. Life Sci 25:2149–2162, 1979

Redmond DE, Katz MM, Maas JW, et al: Cerebrospinal fluid amine metabolites: relationships with behavioral measurements in depressed, manic, and healthy control subjects. Arch Gen Psychiatry 43:938–947, 1986

Remy DC, Rittle KE, Hunt CA, et al: (+)- and (-)-3-methoxycyproheptadine: a comparative evaluation of the antiserotonin, antihistaminic, anticholinergic, and orexigenic properties with cyproheptadine. J Med Chem 20:1681–1684, 1977

Rickels K, Weisman K, Norstad N, et al: Buspirone and diazepam in anxiety: a controlled study. J Clin Psychiatry 43:81–86, 1982

Robichaud RC, Sledge KL: The effects of p-chlorophenylalanine on experimentally induced conflict in the rat. Life Sci 8:965–969, 1969

Ross CA, Matas M: A clinical trial of buspirone and diazepam in the treatment of generalized anxiety disorder. Can J Psychiatry 32:351–355, 1987

Rydin E, Schalling D, Åsberg M: Rorschach ratings in depressed and suicidal patients with low CSF 5-HIAA. Psychiatry Res 7:229–243, 1982

Sanders-Bush E, Breeding M: Putative selective 5-HT$_2$ antagonists block serotonin 5-HT$_{1c}$ receptors in the choroid plexus. J Pharmacol Exp Ther 247:169–173, 1988

Schoeffter PH, Waeber C, Palacios JM, et al: The 5-HT$_{1d}$ receptor subtype is negatively coupled to adenylate cyclase in calf substantia nigra. Naunyn Schmiedebergs Arch Pharmacol 337:602–608, 1988

Sepinwall J, Cook L: Behavioral pharmacology of antianxiety drugs, in Handbook of Psychopharmacology. Edited by Iversen LL, Iversen SD, Snyder SH. New York, Plenum, 1978, pp 345–393

Sheehan DV, Raj AB, Sheehan H, et al: The relative efficacy of buspirone, imipramine and placebo in panic disorder: a preliminary report. Pharmacol Biochem Behav 29:815–817, 1988

Shephard RA, Buxton DA, Broadhurst PL: Drug interactions do not support reduction in serotonin turnover as the mechanism of action of benzodiazepines. Neuropharmacology 21:1027–1032, 1982

Smith TM, Suckow RF: Trazodone and m-chlorophenylpiperazine: concentration in brain and receptor activity in regions in the brain associated with anxiety. Neuropharmacology 24:1067–1071, 1985

Stein L, Wise CD, Berger BD: Antianxiety action of benzodiazepines: decrease in activity of serotonin neurones in the punishment system, in The Benzodiazepines. Edited by Garratini S, Mussini E, Randall LO. New York, Raven, 1973, pp 299–326

Stein L, Wise CD, Belluzzi JD: Effects of benzodiazepines on central serotonergic mechanisms, in Mechanism of Action of Benzodiazepines. Edited by Costa E. New York, Raven, 1975, pp 29–44

Stern RS, Marks IM, Mawson D: Clomipramine and exposure for compulsive rituals: plasma levels, side effects, and outcome. Br J Psychiatry 136:161–166, 1980

Targum SD, Marshall LE: Fenfluramine provocation of anxiety in patients with panic disorder. Psychiatry Res 28:295–306, 1989

Thiebot MH, Hamon M, Soubrie P: Attenuation of induced-anxiety in rats by chlordiazepoxide: role of raphe dorsalis benzodiazepine binding sites and serotonergic neurons. Neuroscience 7:2287–2294, 1982

Thorén P, Åsberg M, Cronholm B, et al: Clomipramine treatment of obsessive-compulsive disorder, I: a controlled clinical trial. Arch Gen Psychiatry 37:1281–1289, 1980a

Thorén P, Åsberg M, Bertilsson L, et al: Clomipramine treatment of obsessive-compulsive disorder, II: biochemical aspects. Arch Gen Psychiatry 37:1289–1295, 1980b

Trulson ME, Arasteh K: Buspirone decreases the activity of 5-hydroxytryptamine-containing dorsal raphe neurons in-vitro. J Pharm Pharmacol 38:380–382, 1985

Tye NC, Everitt BJ, Iversen SD: 5-Hydroxytryptamine and punishment. Nature 268:741–742, 1977

Tye NC, Iversen SD, Green AR: The effects of benzodiazepines and serotonergic manipulations on punished responding. Neuropharmacology 18:689–695, 1979

Van der Maelen CP, Wildeman RC: Ionophoretic and systemic administration of the non-benzodiazepine anxiolytic drug buspirone causes inhibition of serotonergic dorsal raphe neurons in rats (abstract). Fed Proc 43:947, 1984

van Praag HM: Biological suicide research: outcome and limitations. Biol Psychiatry 21:1305–1323, 1986

van Praag HM, Korf J: Endogenous depressions with and without disturbances in 5-hydroxytryptamine metabolism: a biochemical classification? Psychopharmacologia 19:148–152, 1971

van Praag HM, Lemus CZ, Kahn RS: Peripheral hormones: a window on the central MA? Psychopharmacol Bull 22:565–570, 1986

van Praag HM, Asnis GM, Kahn RS, et al: Nosological tunnel vision in biological psychiatry: a place for a functional psychopathology. Ann N Y Acad Sci 600:501–510, 1990

Vogel JR, Beer B, Clody DE: A simple and reliable conflict procedure for testing antianxiety agents. Psychopharmacology (Berlin) 21:1–7, 1971

Volavka J, Neziroglu F, Yaryuria-Tobias JA: Clomipramine and imipramine in obsessive-compulsive disorder. Psychiatry Res 14:83–91, 1985

Waeber C, Scoeffter P, Palacios JM, et al: Molecular pharmacology of 5-HT$_{1d}$ recognition sites: radioligand binding studies in human, pig and calf brain membranes. Naunyn Schmiedebergs Arch Pharmacol 337:595–601, 1988

Wheatley D: Buspirone: multicenter efficacy study. J Clin Psychiatry 43:92–94, 1982

Whitton P, Curzon G: Anxiogenic-like effect of infusing 1-(3-chlorophenyl)piperazine (mCPP) into the hippocampus. Psychopharmacology (Berlin) 100:138–140, 1990

Willoughby JO, Menadue MF, Leibelt HJ: Activation of 5-HT$_1$ serotonin receptors in the medial basal hypothalamus stimulates prolactin secretion in the unaesthetized rat. Neuroendocrinology 47:83–87, 1988

Winter JC: Comparison of chlordiazepoxide, methysergide and cinanserin as modifiers of punished behavior and as antagonists of N,N-dimethyltryptamine. Archives Internationales de Pharmacodynamie 197:147–159, 1972

Wise CD, Berger BD, Stein L: Benzodiazepines: anxiety-reducing activity by reduction of serotonin turnover in the brain. Science 17:181, 1972

Zohar J, Insel TR: Obsessive-compulsive disorder: psychobiological approaches to diagnosis, treatment and pathophysiology. Biol Psychiatry 22:667–687, 1987

Zohar J, Mueller EA, Insel TR et al: Serotonergic responsivity in obsessive-compulsive disorder: comparison of patients and healthy controls. Arch Gen Psychiatry 44:946–951, 1987

Zohar J, Insel TR, Zohar-Kadouch RC, et al: Serotonergic responsivity in obsessive-compulsive disorder: effects of chronic clomipramine treatment. Arch Gen Psychiatry 45:167–172, 1988

Chapter 3

The Role of Corticotropin-Releasing Factor in the Pathophysiology of Anxiety Disorders

Catherine Pihoker, M.D., and
Charles B. Nemeroff, M.D., Ph.D.

A ll higher organisms, including humans, are equipped to deal with perturbations of the environment. Biochemical and behavioral adaptations ensue. There is a state of heightened awareness in which heart rate increases and blood pressure rises, blood sugar rises, and blood is shunted to muscles to improve the odds of escape. This concept, though appreciated for centuries by scientists and nonscientists alike, was aptly labeled by Hans Selye in 1936 as the "stress response." In recent years neuroscientists have begun to elucidate the behavioral, neuroendocrinological, and neurochemical events underlying the stress response.

Anxiety is a feature of the stress response. The physiological and behavioral components of stress and anxiety are enmeshed; both result in a state of heightened vigilance. Sympathoadrenal stimulation results in tachycardia and increases in blood pressure. Decreases in food consumption and sexual activity also occur. Anxiety per se is not necessarily detrimental. Rather, it is a protective "fight or flight" response that occurs in all mammals.

Supported by National Institute of Mental Health Grants MH-42088 and MH-19109, and by a pilot project research grant from The John D. and Catherine T. MacArthur Foundation Mental Health Research Network I (Psychobiology of Depression).

In a general sense the distinction between an appropriate stress response and an anxiety disorder lies in the inciting event or lack thereof, and the frequency with which the response occurs. Thus, in an anxiety disorder, one engages in a "fight or flight" response too often or at inappropriate times. It is apparent that a prolonged or frequently occurring state of anxiety or stress would lead to behavioral, biochemical, and cardiovascular events that have adverse effects—for example, hypercortisolemia, hypertension, and tachycardia.

The distinctions between normal stress and various pathological anxiety states are not well defined in terms of clinical presentation, response to therapy, or neurobiological changes. Anxiety disorders are a heterogeneous group, including panic disorder with and without agoraphobia, generalized anxiety disorder (GAD), posttraumatic stress disorder (PTSD), and others. Anxiety disorders and depression often coexist. In fact, the hypothesis has been raised that depression is a result of stress from pathological anxiety (Lesse 1982).

One approach to elucidate the pathophysiological basis of anxiety disorders is to measure physiological changes that occur during anxiety. In this regard, myriad hormones and neurotransmitters have been evaluated. Cortisol, growth hormone, epinephrine, norepinephrine, adenosine, serotonin, and gamma-aminobutyric acid (GABA) are some of the endogenous neuroregulators that have been extensively examined in stress and anxiety states (for review, see Jesberger and Richardson 1985; Shepard 1987). The investigation of neuropeptides in psychiatric disorders has been a more recent development. One of the prime neuropeptides postulated to play a role in anxiety and affective disorders is corticotropin-releasing factor (CRF), the subject of this chapter.

STRUCTURE AND ACTIVITY OF CORTICOTROPIN-RELEASING FACTOR

Although the existence of CRF had been postulated by scientists for many years, the structure of CRF was not elucidated until Vale et al. (1981) demonstrated that the structure of ovine CRF is a 41–amino acid neuropeptide. Over the past decade, CRF has been unequivocally demonstrated to be the major physiological regulator of ACTH (adrenocorticotropin) secretion, ultimately resulting in activation of adrenocortical glucocorticoid synthesis and release. However, actions of CRF are not limited to activation of the hypothalamo-pituitary-adrenocortical (HPA) axis. CRF apparently acts as a neurotransmitter in extrahypothalamic brain areas. CRF and CRF receptors are found heterogeneously distributed in extrahypothalamic brain regions, including the forebrain (i.e., frontal cortex, amygdala, stria terminalis) and brain stem (e.g., locus coeruleus, parabrachial nucleus). This distribution in limbic areas makes it plausible to hypothesize that CRF plays a role in the pathogenesis of anxiety and affective disorders. In the discussion below we describe in further detail the neuroendocrinology of CRF and then provide evidence from laboratory and clinical studies that supports the hypothesis that CRF plays an important role in anxiety disorders.

The stimulation of release of ACTH and other pro-opiomelanocortin derivatives from the anterior pituitary gland by CRF is mediated through activation of adenylate cyclase. ACTH then acts on the adrenal cortex to promote glucocorticoid synthesis and release. There are a number of other neuropeptides with corticotropin-releasing activity, including arginine-vasopressin (AVP), oxytocin, and catecholamines. However, of the substances identified with this activity, CRF is the most potent, both in vivo and in vitro (Negro-Villar et al. 1987).

Our understanding of the synergistic action of CRF and other corticotropin-releasing hormones is enhanced by the study of Brattleboro rats, which are AVP-deficient. These rats exhibit a relatively normal glucocorticoid response to stress (Arimura et al. 1967). However, when the ACTH concentration induced by hypothalamic extracts of Brattleboro rats is measured in vitro, the CRF activity is found to be only 20% of normal (Gillies and Lowry 1979). Despite the fact that CRF is the most powerful secretagogue of ACTH, its efficacy as a hypophysiotropic hormone is significantly enhanced by other neurotransmitters, such as AVP.

In addition to stimulatory influences on ACTH are inhibitory influences such as those exerted by GABA and opioids, which inhibit CRF secretion (for review, see Owens and Nemeroff 1990). ACTH and glucocorticoids also exert negative feedback effects.

Thus, CRF works in concert with other neuropeptides and hormones to regulate ACTH secretion from the pituitary.

Corticotropin-releasing factor is synthesized in the paraventricular nucleus of the hypothalamus and transported down the axon to nerve terminals of the median eminence, from which it is released into the hypothalamo-pituitary portal system. Under basal conditions, CRF is secreted in a pulsatile fashion, with its pulses roughly preceding by minutes pulses of ACTH. Within minutes of exposure to stress, CRF is secreted into the hypophyseal portal system, with subsequent release of ACTH from the pituitary. Plotsky (1987) reported an increase in portal concentrations of CRF, as well as AVP and epinephrine, in rats subjected to graded hemorrhagic stress.

Passive immunoneutralization of CRF with specific antisera partially or completely blocks the ACTH response expected with stressors such as hemorrhage, insulin-induced hypoglycemia, or ether (Bruhn et al. 1984; Gibbs 1986; Plotsky et al. 1985; Rivier and Vale 1983). Using in situ hybridization, CRF messenger RNA (mRNA) has been detected in the paraventricular nucleus of the hypothalamus and has been found to increase after adrenalectomy or stress (Beyer et al. 1988; Harbuz and Lightman 1989; Jingami et al. 1985; Lightman and Young 1988).

LOCALIZATION OF CORTICOTROPIN-RELEASING FACTOR

As noted above, CRF, in addition to its hypophysiotropic role, functions as a neurotransmitter in the brain. Using density-gradient centrifugation and a sensitive and specific radioimmunoassay, CRF has been demonstrated to be preferentially localized in the synaptosomal fraction of rat brain homogenates (Cain et al. 1991). On electron micrographs of both the rat and human median eminence, CRF has been identified by immunohistochemical methods in large neurosecretory granules. Depolarization of brain slices with potassium in vitro results in CRF release that is calcium-dependent (Smith et al. 1986; Suda et al. 1985). Using electrophysiological methods, CRF has been shown to alter the neuronal firing rate of cells in both the hippocampus and the locus coeruleus (Aldenhoff et al. 1983; Siggins et al. 1985; Valentino and Foote 1988; Valentino et al. 1983). This concatenation of results clearly supports the view that CRF fulfills the requisite criteria for neurotransmitter status.

As briefly described earlier, the heterogeneous distribution of CRF in the mammalian central nervous system (CNS) has been demonstrated by both immunohistochemical and radioimmunoassay studies. CRF is most abundant in the hypothalamus, in limbic structures, and in brain-stem nuclei involved in autonomic regulation. More specifically, regions containing CRF neurons include the central nucleus of the amygdala, bed nucleus of the stria terminalis, substantia innominata, septum, preoptic area, locus coeruleus, parabrachial nucleus, and the dorsal vagal complex (Chappell et al. 1986; Merchenthaler et al. 1984; Moga and Gray 1985; Swanson et al. 1983).

Using autoradiography and radioligand binding studies, putative CRF receptors have also been identified in brain sites outside of the hypothalamic-pituitary axis (De Souza and Insel 1990). The relative concentration of CRF receptors, as observed with autoradiography, roughly parallels the distribution of CRF in extrahypothalamic brain sites (De Souza 1987; De Souza and Insel 1990). Thus, the neuropeptide and receptor distribution, taken together with the CRF pathways known to date and the behavioral effects of CRF (see below), supports a role for CRF as the major coordinator of the stress response.

ANXIOGENIC EFFECTS OF CORTICOTROPIN-RELEASING FACTOR

One method to evaluate the effects of any endogenous substance on the CNS is to directly infuse the neuropeptide into the cerebral ventricles or brain parenchyma. This will mimic the high concentration achieved locally after release from nerve terminals. Such data are available for CRF, and the findings support a role for this peptide in the stress response and in anxiety disorders. In rats, intracerebroventricular (icv) administration of CRF produces physiological and behavioral changes characteristic of stress and similar to certain signs and symptoms of depression and anxiety. The sympathoadrenal activation pathognomonic to the stress response is replicated by icv CRF infusion. Thus, both stress and

CRF produce an increase in epinephrine and norepinephrine secretion, increased heart rate and blood pressure, increased plasma glucagon and glucose concentrations, and decreased gastric acid secretion (Brown 1986; Brown et al. 1982; Fisher et al. 1982, 1983; Lenz et al. 1987).

Central administration of CRF in laboratory rats results in an increase in classical anxiogenic behavior. In a familiar environment, icv CRF produces an increase in behavioral arousal, with a dose-dependent increase in locomotion, sniffing, rearing, and grooming (D. R. Britton et al. 1986; K. T. Britton et al. 1986; Sutton et al. 1982; Tazi et al. 1987). In contrast, when the effects of CRF are examined in novel environments, CRF-treated rats are significantly more fearful and anxious. For example, rats receiving icv CRF demonstrate decreased rearing, increased grooming, and decreased crossing into open spaces when placed in a novel environment (e.g., an open field) (Britton et al. 1982). Similar decreases in exploratory behavior are observed in rats given icv CRF and in rats subjected to 30 minutes of restraint stress (Lee et al. 1987). Other behaviors observed in rats treated with centrally administered CRF include decreased sexual activity and decreased feeding (Dunn and Berridge 1990; Krahn et al. 1986; Morley and Levine 1982; Sirinathsinghji 1987).

The finding that these anxiogenic behaviors are not observed after systemic administration of CRF suggests that these behaviors are centrally mediated, and not mediated by activation of the HPA axis. Further evidence that these effects of CRF are independent of endocrine action is the fact that these behaviors are not mimicked by glucocorticoids (D. R. Britton et al. 1986). It is of great interest to note that the CRF antagonist alpha-helical CRF$_{9-41}$, administered centrally, decreases anxiogenic behaviors and also reverses both stress-induced anorexia and the decrease in exploratory behaviors observed with restraint stress (Berridge and Dunn 1987; Krahn et al. 1986). The anxiogenic effects of CRF are also antagonized by benzodiazepine anxiolytics. For example, in the operant conflict test, CRF (0.5 µg given intracerebroventricularly) resulted in an increased sensitivity to aversive events. This effect was reversed by simultaneous administration of systemic chlordiazepoxide; the benzodiazepine alone increased punished responding, as shown in Figure 3–1 (Koob and

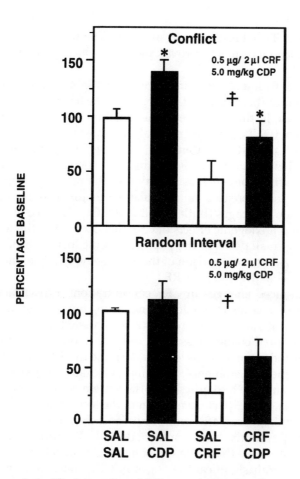

Figure 3–1. The interaction of 0.5 µg corticotropin-releasing factor (CRF) injected intracerebroventricularly and of 5.0 mg/kg chlordiazepoxide (CDP) injected intraperitoneally on responding during the random interval and conflict components of an operant conflict test. Results are expressed as percentage of baseline from the previous day. *Asterisk* denotes significant difference from saline, main effect CDP; double cross denotes significant difference from saline, main effect CRF, *P* < .05, two-way ANOVA. *Source.* Reprinted from Thatcher-Britton K, Morgan J, Rivier J, et al.: "Chlordiazepoxide Attenuates CRF-Induced Responses Suppression in the Conflict Test." *Psychopharmacology* (Berlin) 86:170, 1985. Copyright 1985. Used with permission.

Britton 1990; Thatcher-Britton et al. 1985). The CNS site where CRF produces its anxiety-provoking effects has been investigated.

Bilateral infusion of CRF directly into the locus coeruleus, the site of the noradrenergic cells that project to the forebrain, results in an increase in the norepinephrine metabolite 3,4-dihydroxy-phenylglycol (DHPG) in the amygdala and posterior hypothalamus, which provides evidence of increased norepinephrine turnover. This infusion of CRF into the locus coeruleus results in behavioral activation, such as agitation in the modified Porsolt Swim Test and increased nonambulatory motor activity measured in photocell cages (Butler et al. 1990). Of relevance here is the profound anxiogenic effects of CRF that occur after the infusion of very small doses of the peptide into the locus coeruleus. (See Figure 3–2 for comparison of the anxiogenic effects of intra–locus coeruleus CRF and icv CRF.)

Stress-induced changes in CRF concentration in discrete rat brain regions have also been determined using immobilization at 4°C as an acute stressor. Chronic stress consisted of a 2-week period of unpredictable stressors in order to avoid habituation. Both acute and chronic stress led to a decrease in CRF concentration in the median eminence, presumably because of increased CRF release into the hypophyseal portal system, which activated the HPA axis. The CRF concentration in the locus coeruleus was dramatically increased after both acute and chronic stress. This finding has recently been confirmed by Kalin using stress-induced foot shock (N. Kalin, personal communication, 1990). Other areas with significant changes in CRF concentration included the medial preoptic area (increase with acute stress) and periventricular nucleus of the hypothalamus (increase with chronic stress) (Chappell et al. 1986) (see Figure 3–3).

EFFECTS OF STRESS ON CORTICOTROPIN-RELEASING FACTOR

Stress-induced changes in CRF and POMC mRNAs in the paraventricular nucleus of the hypothalamus and the anterior pituitary gland, respectively, have recently been described. Significant increases in both CRF and POMC mRNAs occurred

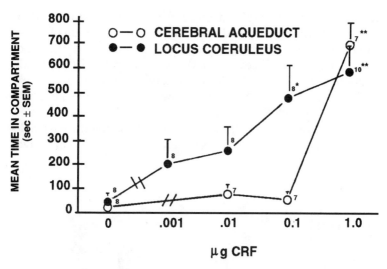

Figure 3–2. Time spent withdrawn in a small, darkened compartment during a 15-minute test period 45 minutes following infusion of corticotropin-releasing factor (CRF) into the cerebral aqueduct or locus coeruleus. The number of animals/group is indicated at each data point. Significantly different from control subjects using Dunnett's test (*$P < .025$, **$P < .001$). *Source.* Reprinted from Butler PD, Weiss JM, Stout JC, et al.: "Corticotropin-Releasing Factor Produces Fear-Enhancing and Behavioral Activation Effects Following Infusion Into the Locus Coeruleus." *Journal of Neuroscience* 10:176–183, 1990. Copyright 1990. Used with permission.

within 4 hours of intraperitoneal hypertonic saline injections. Interestingly, although glucocorticoid (i.e., prednisolone) treatment obliterated the stress-induced increase in POMC mRNA in the anterior pituitary gland, CRF mRNA increases in response to stress persisted despite glucocorticoid treatment (Harbuz and Lightman 1989).

ANXIOLYTICS AND CORTICOTROPIN-RELEASING FACTOR

In laboratory animals, anxiolytics effectively reverse stress-induced behaviors and HPA axis activation. Also, anxiogenic behaviors—for example, decreased social interaction and increased grooming observed with central administration of CRF—can be reversed by antianxiety agents (Dunn and File 1987; Koob and Britton 1990). Because of the integral role of CRF in the endocrinological, autonomic, and behavioral responses to stress, we hypothesized that the effects of the anxiolytic agents might be mediated through CRF neuronal pathways. Two relatively new anxiolytic compounds, alprazolam and adinazolam, are triazolobenzodiazepines. Both have been shown to be effective anxiolytic

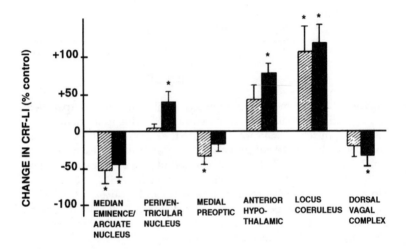

Figure 3–3. Alterations in the concentration of corticotropin-releasing factor (CRF)–like immunoreactivity in brain regions from rats exposed to acute and chronic stress. The hatched bars represent rats exposed to an acute stress, and the solid bars represent rats exposed to chronic (14-day) stress. Values represent percent CRF–like immunoreactivity concentration change in these brain regions relative to control concentrations. Asterisk indicates statistical significance equal to or greater than .05 as determined by ANOVA and Student Newman-Keuls test. *Source.* Reprinted from Bissette G: "Central Nervous System CRF in Stress: Radioimmunoassay Studies," in *Corticotropin-Releasing Factor: Basic and Clinical Studies of a Neuropeptide.* Edited by De Souza EB, Nemeroff CB. Boca Raton, FL, CRC Press, 1990. Copyright 1990. Used with permission.

and antipanic agents. We have evaluated specific changes in regional brain CRF concentrations after acute and chronic alprazolam or adinazolam treatment. Acute alprazolam treatment results in increased hypothalamic CRF concentration and decreased CRF concentration in the locus coeruleus. Both of these effects are opposite to the previously described changes observed after stress (Chappell et al. 1986). Chronic alprazolam treatment results in reduced locus coeruleus CRF concentrations, indicating that there is no tolerance to this effect of the benzodiazepine. Acute withdrawal of alprazolam results in HPA activation, with an increase in plasma ACTH and corticosterone, and decreased amount of anterior pituitary CRF receptor binding. The decrease in pituitary CRF receptor binding is likely due to the downregulation of CRF receptors secondary to CRF hypersecretion. These findings support the hypothesis that CRF mediates certain of the effects of anxiolytic agents such as alprazolam (Owens et al. 1991).

As noted above, intra–locus coeruleus CRF injection produces anxiogenic effects in the rat and increased norepinephrine turnover in brain regions receiving projections from the A6 cell group. Electrophysiological studies have revealed that microinjection of CRF profoundly activates noradrenergic neurons (Valentino et al. 1983). Dunn and Berridge (1987) reported increased noradrenergic turnover in several forebrain structures after icv CRF. These findings, taken together with the well-established observation that agents such as CRF that increase locus coeruleus neuronal activity are anxiogenic, support a role for CRF-norepinephrine interactions in the pathophysiology of anxiety disorders.

Finally, clinical observations have suggested that early stress, trauma, or maternal neglect are associated with an increased incidence of affective and/or anxiety disorders in adulthood. Early stress may lead to long-standing hyperactivity of CRF neurons, perhaps by neuronal sensitization. Significantly increased adrenocortical activity is observed in rats subjected to maternal separation. Our group is presently investigating both hypothalamic and extrahypothalamic CRF neuronal activity and CRF signal transduction in adult rats that have been exposed to repeated maternal separation.

CORTICOTROPIN-RELEASING FACTOR IN PATIENTS WITH ANXIETY DISORDERS

Multiple neuroendocrine and neurotransmitter systems have been scrutinized in patients with anxiety disorders. Overall, the neuroendocrine alterations in patients with anxiety disorders are less striking and reproducible than those observed in patients with major depression (Gold et al. 1987). Reported abnormalities in anxiety disorders include the following: 1) increased basal levels of ACTH and cortisol, 2) blunted thyroid-stimulating hormone and prolactin responses to thyrotropin-releasing hormone administration, and 3) a blunted ACTH but normal cortisol response to CRF (Hollander et al. 1990; Roy-Byrne et al. 1986; Smith et al. 1989). Unlike in major depression, where a significant proportion of patients exhibit cortisol nonsuppression after dexamethasone administration, few patients with anxiety disorders do so (Sheehan et al. 1986). The circadian pattern of cortisol secretion in patients with anxiety disorders appears to be normal. However, the above-mentioned blunted ACTH response to CRF found in patients with panic disorder and patients with PTSD, similar to that observed in patients with affective disorders, suggests intermittent CRF hypersecretion that results in downregulation of CRF receptors in the anterior pituitary.

Over the past decade, substantial evidence has accumulated that suggests a role for CRF in coordinating the endocrinological, autonomic, and behavioral responses to stress. In several psychiatric disorders, including major depression and anorexia nervosa, hyperactivity of CRF neurons has been demonstrated. Although less well studied, the role of CRF in the pathophysiology of anxiety disorders is receiving increasingly more support. Studies of CSF concentrations of CRF in anxiety disorders, particularly during episodes of spontaneous or lactate-induced panic, are needed.

Presently, most of the evidence supporting CRF hyperactivity in patients with anxiety disorders is indirect. In patients with panic disorder, as in patients with depression, the CRF stimulation test results in a blunted ACTH response, suggesting a hyperactive HPA axis. Benzodiazepines, which are effective anxiolytics, have effects on CRF concentration in the brain that are opposite to the effects of stress. Stress-related behaviors are reversed by CRF antagonists. As noted above, more direct studies of CRF activity in patients with anxiety disorders have yet to be performed. These would include measurements of CRF in CSF of treated and untreated patients with anxiety, and of CRF binding studies in postmortem brain tissue. The practical limitations to the study of CNS activity of a neuropeptide, as well as the complex interactions of CRF with other hormones and neurotransmitters, are continual challenges in our study of the involvement of CRF in anxiety disorders. The use of a lipophilic ligand to image brain CRF receptors with positron-emission tomography would be particularly beneficial.

REFERENCES

Aldenhoff JB, Gruol D, Rivier J, et al: Corticotropin-releasing factor decreases post-burst hyper-polarizations and excites hippocampal neurons in vitro. Science 221:875–877, 1983

Arimura A, Saito T, Bowers CY, et al: Pituitary-adrenal activation in rats with hereditary hypothalamic diabetes insipidus. Acta Endocrinol (Copenh) 54:155–165, 1967

Berridge CW, Dunn AJ: A corticotropin-releasing factor antagonist reverses the stress-induced changes of exploratory behavior in mice. Horm Behav 21:393–401, 1987

Beyer HS, Matta SG, Sharp BM: Regulation of the messenger ribonucleic acid for corticotropin-releasing factor in the paraventricular nucleus and other brain sites of the rat. Endocrinology 123:2117–2123, 1988

Britton DR, Koob GF, Rivier J, et al: Intraventricular corticotropin-releasing factor enhances behavioral effects of novelty. Life Sci 31:363–367, 1982

Britton KT, Lee G, Dana R, et al: Activating and "anxiogenic" effects of corticotropin–releasing factor are not inhibited by blockade of the pituitary–adrenal system with dexamethasone. Life Sci 39:1281–1286, 1986

Britton DR, Varela M, Garcia A, et al: Dexamethasone suppresses pituitary-adrenal but not behavioral effects of centrally administered CRF. Life Sci 38:211–216, 1986

Brown M: Corticotropin-releasing factor: central nervous system sites of action. Brain Res 399:10–14, 1986

Brown MR, Fisher LA, Spiess J, et al: Corticotropin-releasing factor: actions on the sympathetic nervous system and metabolism. Endocrinology 111:928–931, 1982

Bruhn TO, Plotsky PM, Vale WW: Effect of paraventricular lesions on corticotropin-releasing factor–like immunoreactivity in the stalk–median eminence: studies on the adrenocorticotropin response to ether stress and exogenous CRF. Endocrinology 114:57, 1984

Butler PD, Weiss JM, Stout JC, et al: Corticotropin-releasing factor produces fear-enhancing and behavioral activation effects following infusion into the locus coeruleus. J Neurosci 10:176–183, 1990

Cain ST, Owens MJ, Nemeroff CB: Subcellular distribution of corticotropin-releasing factor–like immunoreactivity in rat central nervous system. Neuroendocrinology 54:36–41, 1991

Chappell PB, Smith MA, Kilts CD, et al: Alterations in corticotropin-releasing factor–like immunoreactivity in discrete rat brain regions after acute and chronic stress. J Neurosci 6:2908–2914, 1986

De Souza EB: Corticotropin-releasing factor receptors in the rat central nervous system: characterization and regional distribution. J Neurosci 7:88–100, 1987

De Souza EB, Insel TR: Corticotropin-releasing factor (CRF) receptors in the rat central nervous system: autoradiographic localization studies, in Corticotropin-Releasing Factor: Basic and Clinical Studies of a Neuropeptide. Edited by De Souza EB, Nemeroff CB. Boca Raton, FL, CRC Press, 1990

Dunn AJ, Berridge CW: Corticotropin-releasing factor administration elicits a stress-like activation of cerebral catecholaminergic systems. Pharmacol Biochem Behav 27:685–691, 1987

Dunn AJ, Berridge CW: Physiological and behavioral responses to corticotropin-releasing factor administration: is CRF a mediator of anxiety or stress responses? Brain Res Rev 15:71–100, 1990

Dunn AJ, File SE: Corticotropin-releasing factor has an anxiogenic action in the social interaction test. Horm Behav 21:193–202, 1987

Fisher LA, Rivier J, Rivier C, et al: Corticotropin-releasing factor (CRF): central effects on mean arterial pressure and heart rate in rats. Endocrinology 110:2222–2224, 1982

Fisher LA, Jessen G, Brown MR: Corticotropin-releasing factor (CRF): mechanism to elevate mean arterial pressure and heart rate. Regul Pept 5:153–161, 1983

Gibbs DM: Stress-specific modulation of ACTH secretion by oxytocin. Neuroendocrinology 42:97, 1986

Gillies G, Lowry PJ: Corticotropin-releasing factor may be modulated by vasopressin. Nature 278:463–464, 1979

Gold PW, Kling MA, Calabrese JR, et al: Physiological, diagnostic, and pathophysiological implications of corticotropin-releasing hormone, in Handbook of Clinical Psychoneuroendocrinology. Edited by Nemeroff CB, Loosen PT. New York, Guilford, 1987

Harbuz MS, Lightman SL: Responses of hypothalamic and pituitary mRNA to physical and psychological stress in the rat. J Endocrinol 122:705–711, 1989

Hollander E, Levin AP, Liebowitz MR: Biological tests in the differential diagnosis of anxiety disorders, in Clinical Aspects of Panic Disorder. Edited by Ballenger JC. New York, Wiley–AR Liss, 1990

Jesberger JA, Richardson JS: Neurochemical aspects of depression: the past and the future? Int J Neurosci 27:19–47, 1985

Jingami H, Matsukura S, Numa S, et al: Effects of adrenalectomy and dexamethasone administration on the level of preprocorticotropin-releasing factor messenger ribonucleic acid (mRNA) in the hypothalamus and adrenocorticotropin/beta-lipotropin precursor mRNA in the pituitary in rats. Endocrinology 117:1314–1320, 1985

Koob GF, Britton KT: Behavioral effects of corticotropin-releasing factor, in Corticotropin-Releasing Factor: Basic and Clinical Studies of a Neuropeptide. Edited by De Souza EB, Nemeroff CB. Boca Raton, FL, CRC Press, 1990

Krahn DD, Gosnell BA, Grace M, et al: CRF antagonist partially reverses CRF- and stress-induced effects on feeding. Brain Res Bull 17:285–289, 1986

Lee EHY, Tang YP, Chai CT: Stress and corticotropin-releasing factor potentiate center region activity of mice in an open field. Psychopharmacology (Berlin) 93:320–324, 1987

Lenz HJ, Raedler A, Greten H, et al: CRF initiates biological actions within the brain that are observed in response to stress. Am J Physiol 252:R34–R39, 1987

Lesse S: The relationship of anxiety to depression. Am J Psychother 36:332–348, 1982

Lightman SL, Young WS III: Corticotropin-releasing factor, vasopressin and pro-opiomelanocortin mRNA responses to stress and opiates in the rat. J Physiol (Lond) 403:511–523, 1988

Merchenthaler I, Vigh S, Schally AV, et al: Immunocytochemical localization of corticotropin-releasing factor (CRF)–like immunoreactivity in the thalamus of the rat. Brain Res 323:119–122, 1984

Moga MM, Gray TS: Evidence for corticotropin-releasing factor, neurotensin and somatostatin in the neural pathway from the central nucleus of the amygdala to the parabrachial nucleus. J Comp Neurol 241:275–284, 1985

Morley JE, Levine AS: Corticotropin-releasing factor, grooming and ingestive behavior. Life Sci 31:1459–1464, 1982

Negro-Villar A, Johnston C, Spinedi E, et al: Physiological role of peptides and amines on the regulation of ACTH secretion. Ann N Y Acad Sci 512:218–236, 1987

Owens MJ, Nemeroff CB: Neurotransmitter regulation of CRF secretion in vitro, in Corticotropin-Releasing Factor: Basic and Clinical Studies of a Neuropeptide. Edited by De Souza EB, Nemeroff CB. Boca Raton, FL, CRC Press, 1990, pp 107–114

Owens MJ, Bissette G, Nemeroff CB: Acute effects of alprazolam and adinazolam on the concentrations of corticotropin-releasing factor in rat brain. Synapse 4:196–202, 1989

Owens MJ, Vargas MA, Knight DL, et al: The effects of alprazolam on corticotropin-releasing factor neurons in the rat brain: acute time course, chronic treatment and abrupt withdrawal. J Pharmacol Exp Ther 258:349–356, 1991

Plotsky PM: Regulation of hypophysiotropic factors mediating ACTH secretion, in The Hypothalamic-Pituitary-Adrenal Axis Revisited. Ann N Y Acad Sci 512:205–217, 1987

Plotsky PM, Bruhn TO, Vale W: Hypophysiotropic regulation of adrenocorticotropin secretion in response to insulin-induced hypoglycemia. Endocrinology 114:323–329, 1985

Rivier C, Vale W: Modulation of stress-induced ACTH release by corticotropin-releasing factor, catecholamines and vasopressin. Nature 305:325, 1983

Roy-Byrne PP, Uhde TW, Rubinow DR, et al: Reduced TSH and prolactin responses to TRH in patients with panic disorder. Am J Psychiatry 143:503–507, 1986

Selye H: Thymus and adrenals in the response of the organism to injuries and intoxications. Br J Exp Pathol 17:234–248, 1936

Sheehan DV, Claycomb JB, Surman OS, et al: Panic attacks and the dexamethasone suppression test. Am J Psychiatry 140:1063–1064, 1986

Shepard RA: Behavioral effects of GABA agonists in relation to anxiety and benzodiazepine action. Life Sci 40:2429–2436, 1987

Siggins GR, Gruol D, Aldenhoff J, et al: Electrophysiological actions of corticotropin-releasing factor in the central nervous system. Federation Proceedings 44:237–242, 1985

Sirinathsinghji DJS: Inhibitory influence of corticotropin-releasing factor on components of sexual behavior in the male rat. Brain Res 407:185–190, 1987

Smith MA, Bissette G, Slotkin TA, et al: Release of corticotropin-releasing factor from rat brain regions in vitro. Endocrinology 118:1997–2001, 1986

Smith MA, Davidson J, Ritchie JC, et al: The corticotropin-releasing hormone test in post-traumatic stress disorder. Biol Psychiatry 26:349–355, 1989

Suda T, Yajima F, Tomori N, et al: In vitro study of immunoreactive corticotropin-releasing factor release from the rat hypothalamus. Life Sci 37:1499–1504, 1985

Sutton RE, Koob GF, Le Moal M, et al: Corticotropin-releasing factor produces behavioral activation in rats. Nature 297:331–333, 1982

Swanson LW, Sawchenko PE, Rivier J, et al: Organization of ovine corticotropin-releasing factor immunoreactive cells and fibers in the rat brain: an immunohistochemical study. Neuroendocrinology 36:165–186, 1983

Tazi A, Swerdlow NR, Le Moal M, et al: Behavioral activation by CRF: evidence for the involvement of the ventral forebrain. Life Sci 41:41–49, 1987

Thatcher-Britton K, Morgan J, Rivier J, et al: Chlordiazepoxide attenuates CRF-induced responses suppression in the conflict test. Psychopharmacology (Berlin) 86:170–174, 1985

Vale W, Spiess J, Rivier C, et al: Characterization of a 41-residue ovine hypothalamic peptide that stimulates secretion of corticotropin and ß-endorphin. Science 213:1394–1397, 1981

Valentino RJ, Foote SL: Corticotropin-releasing hormone increases tonic but not sensory-evoked activity of noradrenergic locus coeruleus neurons in unanesthetized rats. J Neurosci 8:1016–1025, 1988

Valentino RJ, Roote SL, Aston-Jones G: Corticotropin-releasing factor activates noradrenergic neurons of the locus coeruleus. Brain Res 270:363–367, 1983

Chapter 4

Implications of Cocaine Kindling, Induction of the Proto-oncogene c-fos, and Contingent Tolerance

**R. M. Post, M.D., S. R. B. Weiss, Ph.D.,
T. W. Uhde, M.D., M. Clark, Ph.D., and
J. B. Rosen, Ph.D.**

T he evolution of cocaine-related panic attacks appears to follow a time course that is highly similar to that observed with the pharmacological kindling of cocaine-related seizures. Panic attacks do not usually occur with the initial cocaine administration but may develop over time after many repetitions. Following sufficient episodes of cocaine-related panic attacks, the emergence of panic attacks independent of the use of cocaine can occur—that is, these attacks can become spontaneous. Thus, the study of the evolution of cocaine-related panic attacks may illuminate how a process may emerge and change over time from one that is stimulus precipitated to one that is spontaneous.

The cocaine kindling model for panic attacks also allows focus on what may be important aspects of panic disorder: its evolution over time and the corresponding changes in its biological, neuroanatomic, and pharmacological substrates. The kindling model also permits the analysis of mechanisms that may be in-

This chapter is based in part on a presentation at the annual meeting of the American Psychiatric Association, New York, May 1990.

volved in long-lasting changes in responsivity to pharmacological agents or panicogenic stimuli. For example, the induction of proto-oncogenes, which affect the organism at the level of gene expression, may be one mechanism by which these long-lasting changes can be encoded.

Finally, we describe another preclinical kindling model in which we observed contingent tolerance to the anticonvulsant effects of carbamazepine on amygdala-kindled seizures. This tolerance is not related to pharmacokinetic variables but to the temporal pairing (i.e., contingencies) of drug administration and kindled seizure induction. When the drug and seizure are unpaired (e.g., by administering the drug after the kindled seizure has occurred), not only does tolerance not develop but it may also be reversed because of this change in temporal contingencies. Similar contingent-tolerance mechanisms have been described for benzodiazepines (Mana and Pinel 1990). These data raise the possibility that associative (i.e., learned) variables may be important to consider in the development of refractoriness to the anxiolytic or other therapeutic effects of psychotropic and/or anticonvulsant drugs, and that a potential reversal of this phenomenon can be accomplished by techniques that disrupt the association (e.g., a period of time off medications).

In each of the points discussed in this chapter, potential important clinical implications are raised by new findings in preclinical models. The basic research paradigms may be of considerable importance in answering mechanistic questions related to the phenomena described, as well as in propelling further systematic research on the potential relevance of these findings to principles in the clinical situation. While much direct cross-comparison remains to be conducted in order to assess the applicability of these models to the clinical situation, the current data are presented for their potential heuristic value and in an attempt to encourage further studies in a systematic fashion.

KINDLING OF COCAINE-RELATED PANIC DISORDER

In taking detailed histories of the onset of panic attacks in patients entering a clinical research unit for the study and treatment of panic disorder, Uhde and associates[1] uncovered a number of patients with cocaine-related panic. These data are consistent with the reports by Washton and Gold (1984) that panic attacks are reported in approximately 50% of patients calling a cocaine hotline in order to obtain information and referral regarding treatment for cocaine-related problems. The epidemiological data of Anthony et al. (1989) further confirm the association of cocaine use and panic attacks. In these authors' study, interviewees with a history of cocaine use were 13 times more likely to report panic attacks than were those without a history of cocaine use. Moreover, Aronson and Craig (1986) have recently reported a series of three cases among 60 patients in their clinic in whom the first panic attacks were closely associated with cocaine use.

We present below a detailed case history of the relationship of the development of panic attacks to cocaine use and discuss the possibility that behavioral sensitization and/or kindling-like mechanisms might be relevant to the etiopathogenesis of the development of panic attacks in this and other individuals. Following this, several other cases and series have been reported that are consistent with this kindling formulation (Aronson and Craig 1986; Louie et al. 1989).

Behavioral sensitization involves the increased locomotor or stereotypic response to repeated doses of a psychomotor stimulant or dopamine agonist (Post and Contel 1983). Catecholaminergic mechanisms are implicated in behavioral sensitization. Conditioning plays an important role in cocaine-induced behavioral sensitization (Post et al. 1987b; Weiss et al. 1987, 1989a) and could provide one mechanism for the development of greater, rather than lesser, responsivity to cocaine over time that is observed with the late occurrence of panic attacks. One might then also expect conditioned cues to become increasingly important in precipitating cocaine-related panic attacks.

Pharmacological kindling has been demonstrated with local-

---

[1] This case was initially presented at the meeting of the American College of Neuropsychopharmacology (Post et al. 1986c) and published in 1986 (Post et al. 1986b); it thus represents the first report of the evolution of cocaine-induced panic attacks that follow a kindling-like time course.

anesthetic agents in animals, most notably with lidocaine, which is equipotent to cocaine as a local anesthetic but is not a psycho-motor stimulant (Post et al. 1975, 1984a, 1987a). Thus, repeated administration of the same dose of lidocaine (65 mg/kg ip), which produces no effect for the first several days to weeks of treatment, eventually produces seizures in some animals (Post et al. 1975, 1984a, 1987a). This finding is similar to what is observed with direct electrical stimulation of various brain structures, or "kindling," as originally described by Goddard et al. (1969). They stimulated the amygdala once a day for 1 second, producing an increasing duration and spread of afterdischarges and, finally, the emergence of major motor seizures to previously subthresh-old stimulation (Figure 4–1). This change in excitability is long lasting, as animals that are not stimulated for weeks or months

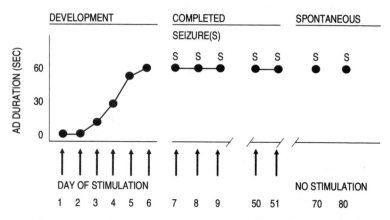

Figure 4–1. Phases of kindling evolution. Three stages can be distinguished: 1) a *development phase* during which time the afterdischarge (AD) threshold decreases, the AD duration becomes longer and more widespread, and partial seizures (behavioral arrest and head nodding; stages 1 and 2) evolve to generalized major motor seizures (involving head, trunk, and forepaws with rearing and falling; stages 4 and 5); 2) a *completed phase* in which a major motor seizure(s) is reliably elicited with each stimulation; and 3) a *spontaneous seizure phase* in which exogenous stimulation is no longer necessary. Stimulation of the amygdala in our studies is given once daily for 1 second (*arrow*) at 60 Hz and 800 µA.

continue to show a full-blown response when finally restimulated (Racine 1972). If kindled animals are subjected to enough seizures, they develop a spontaneous epileptic process in which exogenous physiological stimulation is no longer required (Pinel 1981; Wada et al. 1974). We have also observed "spontaneity" after repeated lidocaine-induced seizures (N. R. Contel, unpublished observations, 1982; S. R. B. Weiss, unpublished observations, 1989) but thus far not after cocaine-induced seizures, because almost all of the rats die after their first or second cocaine-related seizure. Thus, kindling (either electrical or pharmacological) evolves through three general phases: 1) early or developmental (emergence of seizure); 2) mid or completed (reliable seizure induction); and 3) late or spontaneous (exogenous stimulus not required) (see Figure 4–1).

A kindling-like process would provide an explanation for the sudden eruption of a behavioral response—in this case, panic attacks rather than a seizure—to a stimulus that was initially without effect. It could also be used to explain the evolution from drug-related to spontaneous panic attacks following sufficient repetitions of the drug-induced variety. Carbamazepine blocks the development of cocaine- or lidocaine-kindled seizures, but it does not block behavioral sensitization to cocaine's psychomotor stimulant effects (Weiss et al. 1989b, 1990). Thus, a prophylactic response to carbamazepine in the development of cocaine-induced panic attacks would implicate a local anesthetic kindling mechanism.

We now present a case study of a patient with a kindling-like evolution of panic attack as the backdrop for further discussion of the potential clinical implications and mechanisms involved (Post et al. 1986b, 1987a).

Case Study

The patient was a 24-year-old male who presented to the clinic with an approximately 2-year history of panic attacks. He had no psychiatric difficulties prior to 1981, and he had a positive family history of depression and alcoholism but not of panic attacks. His early developmental history and past medical history were unremarkable except for recreational use of alcohol and marijuana. In 1978, at age 19, the patient began to use cocaine intranasally. He also occasionally used ethanol, marijuana, and barbiturates. He continued to use cocaine on an essentially daily basis for approximately 3 years without major untoward side effects. He typically experienced a cocaine-induced rush with feelings of euphoria. In January 1981, he experienced his first cocaine-related panic attack approximately 30 to 45 minutes after sniffing cocaine. This was characterized by a sensation of pressure in his abdomen, chest pain with radiation into his left arm, terror, diaphoresis, hot flashes, and shortness of breath. [This first phase of panic disorder emergence appeared to be highly analogous to the development phase of kindling during which a previously nonconvulsive stimulus comes to evoke a full-blown seizure; in a parallel fashion, panic attacks emerged following a great many cocaine self-administrations.]

Cocaine-induced panic attacks continued to occur, not with every ingestion of cocaine, but on an approximately five-times-per-week basis over the next 6 months. These attacks were associated with only mild agoraphobia and mild generalized anxiety, as the patient linked these panic reactions to the direct effects of cocaine. [This is analogous to the mid or completed phase of kindling.] However, in July 1982, the patient experienced his first spontaneous panic attack (i.e., unrelated to cocaine ingestion). This panic attack was noteworthy in that it was associated with a new and more severe set of symptoms. Gastrointestinal symptoms associated with panic attacks also became more prominent and included abdominal pain with belching, flatulence, hot flashes with diaphoresis, and a sense of impending doom. Progressively more incapacitating agoraphobia also developed as the patient became acutely aware that his panic attacks were no longer closely related to cocaine ingestion and were now unpredictable. Increasingly, the patient was afraid to leave his home area and was unable to travel without the support of a companion. In addition, a higher level of generalized anxiety occurred, and in August and September of 1981, depression severe enough to meet DSM-III criteria was also evident for approximately 1 month. [As these initially cocaine-related panic attacks continued to recur in the absence of cocaine use, they closely conformed to the late, or spontaneous, phase of kindling (Figure 4–1).]

The now spontaneous panic attacks ran an atypical course in terms of psychopharmacological responsivity. The patient showed a fair antipanic response to alprazolam, carbamazepine, and imipramine; however, the response to each of these agents was not complete and the patient remained at least partially symptomatic, continuing to display high levels of generalized anxiety and moderate to severe degrees of agoraphobia. Only following imipramine did the patient's agoraphobia reach a mild baseline.

The course of illness in this patient is similar to that of the three patients who had cocaine-induced panic attacks as described by Aronson and Craig (1986) and the seven patients described by Louie et al. (1989). In our patient and in those described by Louie et al., panic attacks developed as a late consequence of repeated cocaine use, and only after a period of extensive recurrence did they become spontaneous. Family history was negative for panic in all cases. In contrast to our patient, those of Louie et al. (1989) were poorly responsive to traditional tricyclic antidepressant antipanic therapy, but they did respond to alprazolam or carbamazepine.

Our case (Post et al. 1986b) and those of Aronson and Craig (1986) and Louie et al. (1989), along with the epidemiological data of Anthony et al. (1989), suggest that not only may a substantial number of patients experience their first panic attack during cocaine administration, but, in some instances, this process may eventually lead to the development of "spontaneous" panic attacks. The initial mechanisms of the cocaine-induced panic attack, as well as the possible mechanisms that account for its evolution into "spontaneity," are of theoretical as well as practical interest.

Acute Catecholaminergic Mechanisms

Cocaine is a potent blocker of reuptake of the catecholamines dopamine and norepinephrine, as well as the indoleamine serotonin (Post and Contel 1983; Pitts and Marwah 1987a, 1987b; Ritz et al. 1987). The psychomotor stimulant and reinforcing properties of cocaine are thought to be closely associated with catecholamine reuptake blockade and, in particular, with dopamine. For example, large selective depletions of dopamine in the nucleus accumbens block cocaine-induced locomotor hyperactivity in animals (Kelly and Iversen 1976) and also block intravenous cocaine self-administration (Roberts et al. 1980). The prefrontal cortex is also thought to be important in the reinforcing properties of cocaine, since rats will self-administer cocaine directly into this area (Goeders and Smith 1983). Finally, there is a significant correlation between the potencies of cocaine analogs in binding to the dopamine uptake site and their reinforcement efficacy as measured by self-administration procedures in animals (Ritz et al. 1987).

The catecholaminergic potentiating properties of cocaine are of particular interest in relationship to catecholamine theories of the panic anxiety disorders (Charney and Heninger 1985; Redmond and Huang 1979; Uhde et al. 1984). While cocaine acutely inhibits firing of noradrenergic neurons in the locus coeruleus, dopaminergic neurons in the substantia nigra, and serotonergic neurons in the raphe nuclei (Pitts and Marwah 1987a, 1987b), it increases norepinephrine and dopamine at postsynaptic sites, which may be a potential factor in the induction of anxiety and panic.

In this regard, it is also important to consider the incidence of anxiety and panic disorders following the use of other psychomotor stimulants such as amphetamine and methylphenidate. We are not aware of reports of as high an incidence of panic attacks in subjects abusing the closely related but nonlocal-anesthetic psychomotor stimulants amphetamine and methylphenidate (Angrist and Gershon 1970; Connell and Akkerhuis 1958; Ellinwood 1972) as is found in subjects self-referred for cocaine-related difficulties (roughly 50%) (Washton and Tatarsky 1984). To the extent that the psychomotor stimulant properties of these two agents are highly similar and a clinical difference can be demonstrated in the incidence of panic attacks, noncatecholamine mechanisms would be implicated in the evolution of panic attacks (e.g., the local-anesthetic mechanisms of cocaine's actions). An increased incidence of cocaine-induced dysphoria and panic compared with that observed on other psychomotor stimulants is also consistent with the anecdotal literature; cocaine tends to be more often administered in conjunction with heroin (speedballing) in order to dampen the former's anxiogenic effects (Gawin and Ellinwood 1988, 1989; Goodman and Gilman 1970; Washton and Gold 1986). High doses of cocaine are also discriminated by animals as being similar to the anxiogenic cues of the convulsant pentylenetetrazole (Wood and Lal 1987), while lower doses generalize to amphetamine (Emmett-Oglesby et al. 1983). The generalization to pentylenetetrazole implicates noncatecholaminergic effects of cocaine in this anxiety cue.

Acute Local-Anesthetic Effects

The local-anesthetic effects of cocaine could provide an alternative to a catecholaminergic mechanism for cocaine-related panic. We have found that acute intravenous administration of the local anesthetic procaine is capable of inducing a wide range of mood changes (euphoria to panic-like dysphoria) in patients with affective disorders or borderline personality disorder and normal volunteers (Kellner et al. 1987). These dysphoric and panic-like reactions appear to be more likely to occur in the patients compared with the control populations, and especially in those patients with higher initial baseline levels of depression and anxiety.

Increased Responsivity to Cocaine With Chronic Administration

Thus, it is possible that either the acute effects of catecholamine potentiation or the local-anesthetic effects of cocaine could be related to cocaine's ability to induce anxiety and panic. How might these effects relate to the observations typified in the case reported above (also see Figure 4–2) that an extended period of chronic or repetitive administration of cocaine is required prior to the first panic attack and that cocaine-induced panic attacks may then progress to the point at which they occur spontaneously? Two potential mechanisms are discussed below. Behavioral sensitization, which involves increased behavioral responsivity to the same, even low, dose of a stimulant implicates a catecholaminergic mechanism. Pharmacological kindling, in which repeated administration of high but subconvulsive doses of cocaine or lidocaine eventually produces full-blown seizures, implicates a local-anesthetic mechanism.

Behavioral Sensitization

As noted above, in the behavioral sensitization model, the effects of cocaine are highly environmental/context–dependent. That is, animals show increased behavioral responsivity to cocaine (hyperactivity and stereotypy) when they had previously been treated with cocaine in the same environment in which they are being tested (Post et al. 1981, 1987a; Weiss et al. 1990). However, if they had been treated with equal amounts of cocaine in a different environment from where they are tested, behavioral sensitization is not evident (Post et al. 1987b; Weiss et al. 1990).

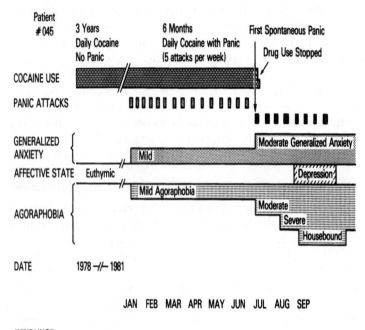

Figure 4-2. The course of development of panic disorder for an individual patient who repeatedly used cocaine *(top bar)* is illustrated. Following 3 years of essentially daily cocaine insufflation by the intranasal route, this patient began to develop panic attacks *(rectangles)* immediately after cocaine, perhaps paralleling the development phase of kindling. Panic attacks occurred approximately 3 times/week for the next 6 months (mid or completed phase). Following these many repetitions of cocaine-induced panic attacks, he developed the first spontaneous panic attack *(shaded rectangle)*, at which time the patient discontinued his cocaine use. Nonetheless, spontaneous panic attacks persisted and the patient developed more severe associated psychiatric symptoms (i.e., generalized anxiety and incapacitating agoraphobia).

These data in animals indicating the importance of conditioning in cocaine-related effects are consistent with a growing body of clinical evidence of the importance of conditioned cues in cocaine-related craving, euphoria, abstinence effects, and relapse (Childress et al. 1987, 1988; Gawin and Ellinwood 1989; Gawin and Kleber 1987).

Although behavioral sensitization and the catecholamine model are attractive candidates for the late induction of increased behavioral response (including panic), there is some clinical and experimental evidence (Fischman et al. 1976, 1983a, 1983b) that tachyphylaxis may develop to the effects on euphoria and blood pressure following repeated administration of the same dose of cocaine, particularly when intervals between doses are short. Moreover, because cocaine's euphorigenic properties have anecdotally been reported to develop some degree of tolerance, subjects tend to increase doses self-administered in order to achieve the same degree of "high." This might be the rationale for dose escalation that allows the local-anesthetic actions of cocaine (achieved at higher concentrations) to come into play. Cocaine abusers have been known to snort, ingest, or inhale 500 to 1,000 mg or more per day on a regular basis.

Local-Anesthetic Kindling: Development, Completed, and Spontaneous Stages

We suggest that the repeated high-dose administration of local anesthetics on an intermittent basis may be associated with a pharmacological kindling effect in which the anxiogenic components of cocaine response are progressively enhanced because of increasing electrophysiological responsivity in deep structures of the brain, particularly the amygdala and hippocampus, and in related limbic structures that are sensitive to the electrophysiological and metabolic effects of the local anesthetics (Post et al. 1975, 1984a, 1984b, 1986c, 1987b). In addition to our observations on the anxiogenic effects of acute administration of the local anesthetic procaine, repeated local-anesthetic use was found to be associated with the development of "doom anxiety" (Saravay et al. 1987).

Analogous to the process of increasing response to repeated

stimulation observed in electrical and pharmacological kindling, the patient in our case example (see above) appears to have developed a behavioral response (panic attacks) to a dose of cocaine that had been administered multiple times over a period of 3 years without such consequences. With sufficient repetition, this cocaine-related pattern eventually led to the development of spontaneous panic attacks, perhaps akin to the process in electrical and pharmacological kindling in which, if kindled seizures are induced often enough, seizures may ultimately begin to occur spontaneously (i.e., without exogenous electrophysiological stimulation.) The patient in the case example (also see Figure 4–2) himself made the link that the "spontaneous" panic attacks were generated by his prior cocaine administration and, realizing this, immediately discontinued his cocaine use. The patient did not feel compelled to stop using the cocaine as long as the panic attacks were closely linked to the cocaine administration. Thus, the spontaneous phase of the panic attacks, as well as the uncertainty about their timing (i.e., unpredictability), appears to have been a particularly anxiety-inducing experience and one that led not only to the patient's discontinuation of cocaine administration but also to the unfolding of associated symptomatology of generalized anxiety and agoraphobia.

In this fashion, we are using the kindling model to suggest that some of the behavioral (if not convulsive) concomitants of repeated cocaine use may increase and evolve over time. We are obviously only drawing an analogy to full-blown kindling of seizures, because panic attacks, and not seizures, were observed in this patient. Panic can be a concomitant of the administration of a variety of compounds at or near the convulsive dose, including cocaine, procaine, pentylenetetrazole, FG 7142, and caffeine, as well as drugs not usually associated with seizures, such as lactate, yohimbine, isoproterenol, *m*-chlorophenylpiperazine, and cholecystokinin (Table 4–1). Anxiety is also one of the most frequent responses to electrical stimulation of the deep temporal lobe structures in humans (Halgren et al. 1978). Local spindles, spikes, and afterdischarges (short of a full-blown seizure) have been documented in humans following use of cocaine (Ellinwood et al. 1977; Stevens et al. 1969) and other local anesthetics (De Jong and Walts 1966).

Kellner et al. (1987) have found that increases in fast activity on the electroencephalogram (EEG) recorded over the temporal lobe are associated with the severity of dysphoria induced by intravenously administered procaine. Thus, it is possible that an excitatory process and increased fast activity (if not a focal after-discharge) could occur and could increase in magnitude upon repetition of local-anesthetic administration in man just as occurs in animals. Electrical and behavioral changes short of seizures are observed to increase over time in both electrical and pharmaco-

Table 4–1.   Panicogenic agents

	Low-dose effect	Mechanism	High-dose convulsant effect	Mechanism
Cocaine	Stimulant (panic)	Dopamine	+++	Local anesthetic
Lidocaine	Nonstimulant (panic)	—	++	Local anesthetic
Procaine	Nonstimulant (panic)	—	++	Local anesthetic
FG 7142	Anxiety, panic	Inverse benzodiazepine agonist	++	Inverse agonist; inhibition of chloride flux
Metrazole	Anxiety, panic	?	++	? Inhibition of chloride flux
Caffeine	Arousal, panic	Adenosine receptor blockade	++	Adenosine A_2 inhibition
Yohimbine	Anxiety, panic	α_2 inhibition firing of locus coeruleus	++	? α_2 inhibition ? inverse benzodiazepine agonist
Isoproterenol	Arousal, panic	β-blockade	?	
m-CPP[a]	Arousal, panic	5-HT$_{(\ )}$ receptor agonist	?	
Cholecystokinin (CKK)	Arousal, panic	Co-transmitter peptide with dopamine or GABA[b]	?	
Lactate	Anxiety, panic	?	?	

[a]*m*-Chlorophenylpiperazine.
[b]Gamma-aminobutyric acid.

logical kindling studies in animals. For example, afterdischarge thresholds progressively decrease and afterdischarge durations increase in electrical kindling, both of which may be behaviorally relevant (Adamec 1975). Abnormal behaviors such as omniphagia may also progressively increase following repeated local-anesthetic administration that does not result in seizures (Post et al. 1975).

Although seizures did not occur in our patient, 7% of the patients calling the cocaine hotline reported cocaine-induced seizures. Cocaine-related seizures are increasingly recognized in the neurologic literature (Alldredge et al. 1989; Lathers et al. 1988; Merriam et al. 1988; Myers and Earnest 1984). These reports include first-onset seizures (Dhuna and Pascual-Leone 1990) and complex partial seizure status (Ogunyemi et al. 1989). The first human case consistent with a kindling-like time course of cocaine seizure evolution has now also been reported (Dhuna and Pascual-Leone 1990). Thus, cocaine kindling to a seizure endpoint has been reported in virtually every species, including rat (Downs and Eddy 1932b), cat (R. M. Post et al., unpublished observations), dog (Downs and Eddy 1932a), rhesus monkey (Post et al. 1976), and humans (Dhuna and Pascual-Leone 1990). It would be expected that some behavioral and affective changes occurring prior to the development of full-blown seizures might also follow a kindling-like time course.

Not only are the spikes in limbic structure observed during cocaine administration consistent with our kindling formulations (Stevens et al. 1969), but also focal increases in glucose utilization in the medial temporal structures, as measured by positron-emission tomography (PET), are observed in several patients with stimulant-induced panic attacks and amnesia when studied in the medication-free state (Baxter et al. 1988). Does this metabolic "hot spot" reflect a kindled focus? Interestingly, these focal increases were partially suppressed by treatment with carbamazepine.

Pharmacological Response: Implications for Differential Mechanisms

Parenterally administered benzodiazepines in animals appear to be potent in inhibiting the development of lidocaine-kindled seizures (Post et al. 1987a). Carbamazepine also effectively inhibits the development of lidocaine- and cocaine-induced kindled seizures (Post et al. 1986d; Weiss et al. 1987, 1989b, 1990) (Figures 4–3 and 4–4). Carbamazepine will not, however, inhibit fully developed lidocaine-kindled seizures (Figure 4–3). Moreover, if acute high doses of cocaine are administered, carbamazepine may actually enhance acute seizures and associated lethality, which is in contrast to its positive effects on cocaine kindling development. These results are opposite to those observed with electrical kindling of the amygdala, in which carbamazepine will not block the development of amygdala-kindled seizures in the rat, but is a highly effective acute anticonvulsant on completed kindled seizures (Figure 4–3). It is noteworthy that diazepam is highly effective in the development and completed stages of amygdala kindling but will not inhibit the later, spontaneous phases (Pinel 1981). In contrast, Pinel (1981) has reported that phenytoin, which is inadequate in the early phases of kindling, is quite good at preventing spontaneous seizures.

These data, summarized in Figure 4–5, suggest the possibility that the pharmacology of cocaine-related panic could also differ in its early stages, when it is closely associated with drug administration, compared with later stages, when it has become spontaneous. The early-development phase of behavioral sensitization is also differentially responsive to neuroleptics when compared with the later expression phase of sensitization (Weiss et al. 1989a). Thus, our data and those in the literature would suggest that different phases of cocaine-induced activation of behavior and anxiety evolution may be differentially responsive to pharmacological agents, particularly if the kindling models are relevant.

Extrapolation from our data in animals would suggest that anticonvulsant benzodiazepines and chronic oral carbamazepine may be effective in preventing the development of cocaine-induced panic attacks to the extent that the pharmacotherapy of these attacks parallels the development of local-anesthetic–kindled seizures. Acute treatment or even repeated intermittent carbamazepine would not be expected to block cocaine-induced panic once this condition has fully developed (see Figures 4–3 and 4–4).

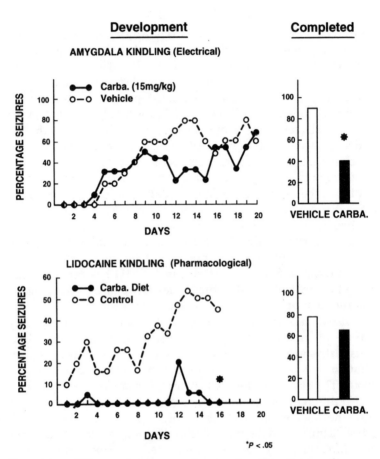

Figure 4–3. Efficacy of carbamazepine as a function of stage of kindling. The early developmental phase of amygdala kindling in the rat is not responsive to carbamazepine (carba.) treatment *(top left)*, whereas the mid phase, wherein seizures are regularly triggered by amygdala stimulation, is very responsive to carbamazepine (also 15 mg/kg ip, *top right; *P < .01*). Conversely, the early developmental phase of pharmacological kindling with lidocaine *(bottom left; *P < .01)* or cocaine (not illustrated) is very responsive to carbamazepine chronically administered in the diet, but carbamazepine in doses of 15 to 50 mg/kg is unable to inhibit completed lidocaine-kindled seizures *(bottom right)* or high-dose acute cocaine seizures (not illustrated). Thus, carbamazepine is effective in some stages of the kindling process but not others, and this varies with different types of kindling.

In relation to blockade of the spontaneous phase of panic attacks in our current patient and in those of Louie et al. (1989), it appeared that these patients were responsive to treatment with

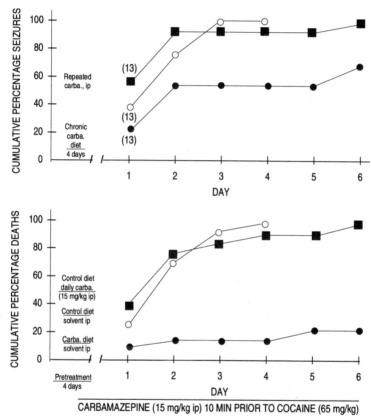

Figure 4–4. Inhibition of cocaine seizures and lethality by carbamazepine. Pretreatment with chronic carbamazepine in diet (not repeated injection) is required to inhibit cocaine seizures and lethality. Rats were treated with chronic carbamazepine in the diet *(closed circles)*, carbamazepine (15 mg/kg ip once daily 10 minutes prior to cocaine) *(closed squares)*, or vehicle *(open circles)* for 4 days prior to cocaine injections and were continued on this regimen throughout the study. The repeated intraperitoneal carbamazepine had no effect on the development of cocaine-kindled seizures or deaths, whereas the chronic carbamazepine inhibited both seizures and deaths.

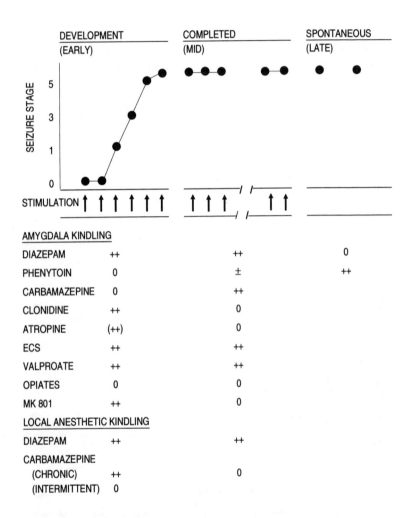

Figure 4–5. Pharmacological responsivity as a function of stage of kindling. Anticonvulsant manipulations are effective in some phases of amygdala kindling but not others. Phases include 1) early (development); 2) mid (completed); and 3) late (spontaneous). Carbamazepine dissociations (see Figure 4–3) are summarized here. While carbamazepine is ineffective (0) on development and highly effective (++) on completed, clonidine, atropine, and the NMDA antagonist MK 801 show the opposite profile. Pinel (1983) documents the efficacy of diazepam early but not late. Phenytoin shows the opposite pattern.

the anticonvulsant alprazolam, which has important actions through the "central-type" benzodiazepine receptor, and with the anticonvulsant carbamazepine, which is thought to exert its anticonvulsant effects, in part, through the "peripheral-type" benzodiazepine receptor (Weiss et al. 1985). Similarly, the tricyclic antidepressant imipramine, even though it is not considered a clinically useful anticonvulsant, was effective in ameliorating the spontaneous panic attacks in our patient and in one of the patients reported by Aronson and Craig (1986). It is noteworthy that some studies have reported that tricyclics will inhibit various phases of amygdala-kindled seizures, particularly when these agents are given acutely (Peterson and Albertson 1982). However, chronically administered desipramine, in doses that, in animals, downregulate ß-adrenergic receptors (10 mg/kg bid), not only failed to block cocaine kindling but actually exacerbated seizure evolution and lethality (Figure 4–6). Moreover, the patients with cocaine-induced panic reported by Louie et al. (1989) were not tricyclic-responsive in their "spontaneous phase."

Theoretical Implications

The evolution of cocaine-related panic attacks from the directly induced form to the spontaneous form appears to provide a unique clinical research opportunity to study the mechanisms underlying this progression of symptomatology. We suggest that components of both the behavioral sensitization and the electrophysiological kindling models are important possible mediators of such a phenomenon. To the extent that behavioral sensitization is relevant for the induction of cocaine-induced panic attacks, it would suggest an important role of conditioning that should be explored in subsequent clinical studies. This phenomenon would tend to implicate catecholaminergic mechanisms in the progressive behavioral changes, especially those in mesolimbic and mesocortical dopamine areas. We postulate an important role for the local-anesthetic component of cocaine's properties, which, with sufficient repetition, could activate kindling-like mechanisms in limbic system structures that are responsible for progressive changes in threshold and excitability. This could lead to the sudden eruption of panic attacks, and, in the ultimate analogy to kindled seizures, repeated cocaine use can actually lead to cocaine-induced seizures (Dhuna and Pascual-Leone

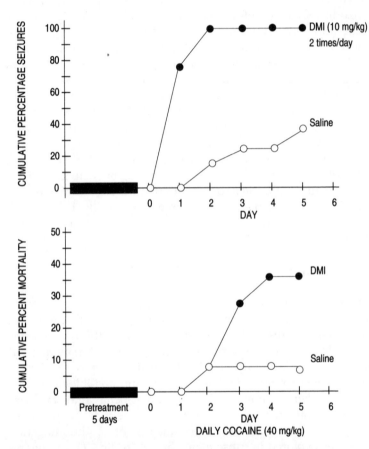

Figure 4–6. Potentiation of cocaine kindling and lethality by the tricyclic antidepressant desipramine (DMI). Not only does desipramine not block the development of cocaine-kindled seizures (open circles) *(top)* or their associated lethality *(bottom)* as does the tricyclic anticonvulsant carbamazepine (see Figure 4–4), but it exacerbates cocaine kindling. This occurs at doses and time courses of desipramine administration (5-day pretreatment and then continuation during cocaine) that are known to downregulate β-adrenergic receptors.

1990). Like kindled seizures, cocaine-related panic attacks may progress to a spontaneous phase.

Response to carbamazepine provides a direct test of the catecholamine-sensitization versus local-anesthetic kindling hypotheses. Carbamazepine does not block acute stimulant motor activation in animals (Post et al. 1984a; Weiss et al. 1990) or euphoria (induced by methylphenidate) in humans (Meyendorff et al. 1985), nor has it been found to block the development of behavioral sensitization to cocaine (Post et al. 1984c, 1988; Weiss et al. 1990). However, it has been shown to block the development of local-anesthetic–kindled seizures (see Figures 4–3 and 4–4). Thus, if carbamazepine blocks the development of cocaine-induced panic attacks, local-anesthetic– rather than catecholamine-mediated psychomotor stimulant effects would be implicated.

Given the report of Baxter et al. (1988) of increased glucose utilization in selective areas of the temporal lobe in stimulant abusers with panic attacks, it may soon be possible to document or disconfirm the kindling hypothesis on the basis of foci of increased metabolic activity in temporal lobe and limbic structures.

Consideration of the role of behavioral sensitization and pharmacological kindling in the development of cocaine-induced panic attacks may lead to new and more specific data gathering and testing of these hypotheses, as well as to more adequate pharmacological intervention, including prophylaxis and treatment of this syndrome. These paradigms may also provide a bridge for considering how non–drug-induced panic syndromes may evolve, particularly since cocaine may share some common substrates with stress effects. Cocaine and stress cross-sensitize to each other with respect to locomotor activity (Antelman 1988; Antelman et al. 1980). Cocaine also releases corticotropin-releasing hormone (CRH) (Calogero et al. 1988; Rivier and Vale 1987), which has been shown to induce limbic seizures following intracerebroventricular administration of high doses (Ehlers et al. 1983; Weiss et al. 1986). Intracerebral or intrathecal administration of endogenous stress–related peptides such as enkephalin and β-endorphin may produce kindling (Cain and Corcoran 1984).

MAPPING THE POTENTIAL NEURAL SUBSTRATES OF PANICOGENIC AGENTS WITH THE PROTO-ONCOGENE *C-FOS*

As summarized in Table 4–1, a variety of convulsant compounds have been reported to induce panic attacks at doses that are subconvulsant. Mapping of the pathways involved in the seizures produced by these agents may thus provide some identification of the putative neural substrates activated. The recently discovered proto-oncogenes *c-fos* and *c-jun* demonstrate rapid mRNA expression within minutes in response to activation of specific neurons and pathways by stressors and seizures. While a number of the panicogens induce proto-oncogenes in common areas of the brain, such as the dentate gyrus of the hippocampus, other agents appear to activate proto-oncogenes in different brain areas. These findings that different seizure subtypes activate different neuronal pathways may be pertinent to our consideration of panic disorder. It is possible that different types of panicogens activate different neural substrates in brain, even if there are some final common pathways, such as the dentate gyrus of the hippocampus, that are also activated.

In the second part of this section, we will raise and discuss the possibility that the induction of proto-oncogenes such as *c-fos* may be more than just a tool for mapping neuronal substrates involved in convulsant reactions and stress. That is, it is possible that with the induction of *c-fos* a series of changes occur, including alterations in gene transcription, which then affect the modification and synthesis of new proteins that might have long-lasting consequences for the organism. In this fashion, it is conceptualized not only that stressors and panicogens may have acute effects on the organism, but via alterations in proto-oncogenes these events may leave behind a long-lasting "memory" of the event, which could affect subsequent reactivity of the organism or the patient.

Proto-oncogenes are normal constituents of cells. At first only the related viral oncogenes were thought to exist. However, once oncogenes were found to be normal cellular constituents, investigation of their role in normal physiological function began. Oncogenes such as *c-fos* and *c-jun* are *transcription factors* (i.e., they affect subsequent gene transcription) and are the earliest genes to be turned on. They are therefore called *immediate-early genes*. Thus, neurotransmitters act as first messengers, and cyclic AMP and related postreceptor events act as second messengers, and now we might conceptualize *c-fos* and related proto-oncogenes as third messengers. These oncogene transcription factors are capable of inducing gene expression, resulting in long-lasting alterations in neurotransmitters, enzymes, peptides, receptors, and even growth factors that may change the structure of synaptic and neural elements.

The proto-oncogene *c-fos* acts as a transcription factor that is induced following activation of neuronal pathways. This induction can be achieved by voltage-dependent calcium influx (Morgan and Curran 1986, 1988, 1989a); by receptor-mediated events—for example, N-methyl-D-aspartate (NMDA) receptors, β_1 receptors, α_1, α_2, acetylcholinergic M_1 receptors, μ receptors, D_1 receptors, vasoactive intestinal peptide (VIP), and adenosine A_2 antagonism (Arenander et al. 1989; Gubits et al. 1989)—and by postreceptor events such as activation of protein kinase C (Shibanuma et al. 1987) or adenylate cyclase (Bravo et al. 1987; Dragunow and Faull 1989; Tramontano et al. 1986).

Given this wide array of molecular events that are capable of inducing *c-fos*, it is not surprising that this oncogene can also be induced by a variety of stimuli and situations that affect neural activity in synaptic transmission. Although we will initially focus on the role of seizures in inducing *c-fos*, most pertinent to the focus of this chapter is the notion that a variety of environmental stressors and subconvulsant stimuli can also induce *c-fos*.

Induction of *c-fos* by Seizures and Stress

As illustrated in Figure 4–7, the pattern of *c-fos* induction following an electroconvulsive seizure (ECS) can be mapped using in situ hybridization. With this technique, a cDNA probe for the proto-oncogene *c-fos* is labeled with ^{35}S, which emits a beta particle that can mark the location of the binding (hybridizing) to the mRNA for *c-fos*. As illustrated in Figure 4–7D, very little *c-fos* is induced in the basal state when animals are not handled or stimulated. In marked contrast (Figure 4–7A), increases in *c-fos* mRNA expression are observed following ECS in the hippocampus, particularly the dentate gyrus and CA-1 hippocampal pyramidal cells; and part of the amygdala complex (e.g., the posterior amygdala cortical nuclei); as well as several septal nuclei bilaterally in mouse brain (Daval et al. 1989; Nakajima et al. 1989c). The piriform cortex and ventral medial nucleus of the hypothalamus are also prominently involved. Interestingly, there may be tolerance to or downregulation of the effect of electroconvulsive shock with chronic administration (Winston et al. 1990). The ear clip control animals (i.e., sham-ECS), illustrated in 4–7B, demonstrate significant increases in c-fos mRNA in the dentate gyrus, the pyramidal cells of the hippocampus, the piriform and other cortical areas, and the cerebellum (Daval et al. 1989).

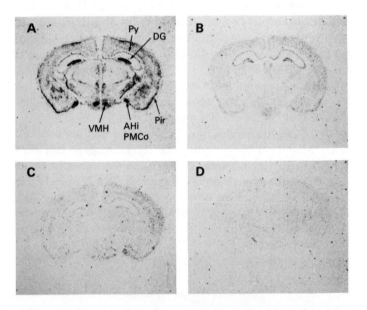

Figure 4–7. In situ hybridization of *c-fos* mRNA in the mouse. Following *(A)* acute electroconvulsive seizure (ECS); *(B)* sham ECS (ear-clip control); *(C)* saline injection; *(D)* no treatment. Abbreviations: Py, pyramidal cells of hippocampus; DG, dentate gyrus; Pir, piriform cortex; AHi, amygdalohippocampal area; PMCo, posteromedial cortical amygdaloid nucleus; VMH, ventromedial hypothalamic nucleus (see Nakajima et al. 1989a for details).

These data suggest that the stress associated with a clothespin–like apparatus applied to the ear in the sham-ECS situation is capable of inducing *c-fos* mRNA. Even very mild stressors appear capable of producing this induction in the mouse, as illustrated by the effects of a single intraperitoneal saline injection (Figure 4–7C) (Nakajima et al. 1989c). These data, which provide the first evidence of stress-induced induction of *c-fos* mRNA in a region-specific fashion, have now been extended using other stressors (Ceccatelli et al. 1989, and others [see below]). These data are also pertinent to the recent findings of Clark and associates (1991b) that the putative stress hormone CRH is capable of inducing *c-fos* mRNA unilaterally in the piriform cortex following intracerebroventricular administration when no seizure occurs. Bilateral *c-fos* induction in the dentate gyrus of the hippocampus was seen in association with a CRH-induced seizure (Figure 4–14).

Thus, physiological stressors (Daval et al. 1989; Nakajima et al. 1989a, 1989c), pharmacological stressors (Ceccatelli et al. 1989; Smith et al. 1991), and nociceptive stimulation as well (Bullitt 1989; Draisci and Iadarola 1989; Hunt et al. 1987) are capable of inducing *c-fos*. It is particularly noteworthy that the piriform cortex is activated by mild stressors or CRH, since this area of the brain has been shown to be involved in the initial phases of amygdala kindling (Burchfiel et al. 1990; Clark et al., 1991a).

Amygdala-Kindled Seizure Evolution Mapped by *c-fos*

During amygdala-kindled seizure evolution, animals progress through different seizure stages that are associated with differential *c-fos* induction:

- Stages 1 and 2: Behavioral arrest and head nodding
- Stage 3: Unilateral forepaw involvement
- Stage 4: Bilateral involvement of the head, trunk, or forepaws
- Stage 5: Bilateral involvement with rearing and falling

The earliest stage-1 and stage-2 amygdala-kindled seizures unilaterally involve either the piriform cortex or the dentate gyrus of the hippocampus. The pattern of *c-fos* induction that was initially elicited (i.e., piriform or dentate gyrus) is dependent on the duration of afterdischarges as recorded from the amygdala (i.e., short or long duration, respectively). Regardless of the initial unilateral *c-fos* pattern at stages 1 and 2, the induction of *c-fos* becomes bilateral with seizure evolution. These data by Clark and associates (1991a) represent the first evidence using the proto-oncogene *c-fos* as a marker for clear-cut, progressive evolution of the anatomic substrates involved in kindling as a function of kindled-seizure stage evolution. Changes are initially unilateral, and they then spread bilaterally to involve greater areas of brain with seizure generalization. These data are convergent with other data mapping the development and progression of electrical afterdischarges with amygdala kindling as well as preliminary data mapping regional changes in glucose utilization. What is unique about the mapping of the neural substrates involved with in situ hybridization is the precision of the technique in conveying the important sense of change in the spatial dimension as a function of time and repeated stimulations.

We also asked whether a similar evolution might occur with pharmacological kindling with cocaine seizures and with a variation on this in the case of cocaine-kindled panic attacks. Repeated subconvulsant administration of cocaine (40 mg/kg ip) produced little evidence of change in *c-fos* mRNA mapped by in situ hybridization. However, when the repeated administration was sufficient to induce a full-blown cocaine-kindled seizure, prominent induction of *c-fos* was observed, not only in the same regions of brain involved with amygdala-kindled seizures (i.e., dentate gyrus of the hippocampus, many cortical areas, and piriform cortex), but in the striatum as well (Clark et al. 1992).

Caffeine-Induced *c-fos* Expression: Striatal Distribution

The data on amygdala kindling and cocaine are particularly noteworthy in relation to the almost exclusive induction of *c-fos* in the striatum in the mouse by the panicogen caffeine. As illustrated in Figures 4–8 and 4–9, inductions of *c-fos* by caffeine were dose related and were prominent at subconvulsant doses of this agent. At all doses of caffeine, the inductions of *c-fos* were largely confined to the striatum and olfactory tubercles (Figure 4–9). Even with the occurrence of caffeine-induced seizures at the highest doses in the mouse, the dentate gyrus of the hippocampus was not involved.

These data suggest that different seizure mechanisms involving different biochemical effects can activate different convulsive pathways in brain. In contrast with the widespread induction of *c-fos* with ECS and cocaine, caffeine inductions were largely confined to striatum, which correlated well with caffeine's blockade of adenosine A_2 receptors (Figure 4–10). The caffeine-induced *c-fos* inductions could be reversed by the adenosine A_2 agonist 5'-N-ethylcarboxamido-adenosine (NECA) but not by the A_1 agonist N^6-cyclohexyladenosine (CHA) (Nakajima et al. 1989b).

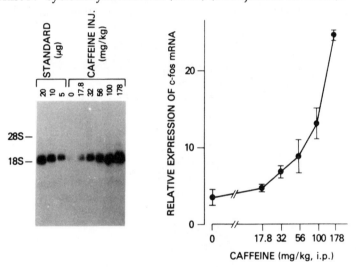

Figure 4–8. Dose response of caffeine-induced *c-fos* mRNA expression in the mouse. In the representative northern blot each number shows the dose of caffeine administration. Fifteen micrograms of each total RNA sample as well as serial-diluted standards were fractionated and hybridized with a ^{32}P-labeled nick-translated mouse *c-fos* DNA probe. The positions of 28S and 18S are indicated as size markers. Reported values are means ± SEM obtained from densitometric scans of northern blots that were separately performed using triplicate samples. Doses 17.8 through 100 mg/kg were subconvulsant; 178 mg/kg produced seizures (see Nakajima et al. 1989b for details).

Caffeine-induced panic attacks have been discussed in detail by Uhde and associates elsewhere (see Uhde 1990). Briefly, it is of considerable interest that Boulenger and Uhde (1982) identified a possible increased sensitivity to the anxiogenic effects of caffeine in panic disorder patients on the basis of preliminary question-naire surveys. They subsequently documented altered sensitivity to panic in panic disorder patients compared with normal volun-teers following double-blind ingestion of caffeine (480 mg) and of placebo. While none of the normal volunteers showed panic at-tacks at this dosage, approximately 40% of the panic disorder patients experienced panic attacks following administration of caffeine (Uhde 1990; Uhde et al. 1990). The panic attacks, which may come in waves, were in many instances virtually identical to

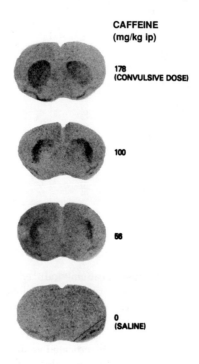

**CAFFEINE
(mg/kg ip)**

178
(CONVULSIVE DOSE)

100

56

0
(SALINE)

Figure 4–9. Dose-dependent *c-fos* expression (0, 56, 100, and 178 mg/kg ip of caffeine and saline) in mouse brain coronal sections shown at the caudate-putamen level.

those experienced by the patients as part of their typical attacks. Subsequent pharmacological studies demonstrated that these attacks were blocked by administration of alprazolam but not imipramine (Uhde and Tancer 1989). In a separate study (see also

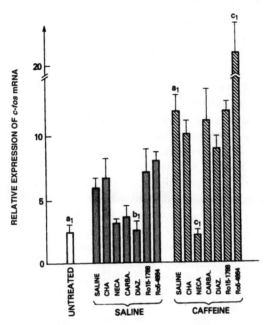

Figure 4–10. Effect of CHA (an A_1 agonist), NECA (an A_2 agonist), carbamazepine, diazepam, Ro 15-1788, and Ro 5-4864 on caffeine-induced *c-fos* expression. Indicated drugs ($n = 4$ in each group) or saline ($n = 8$) were intraperitoneally injected 20 minutes prior to either 100 mg/kg caffeine or saline injection. Each sample, along with serial dilution standards, was loaded in the gels in parallel. Each bar represents the mean relative *c-fos* mRNA expression ± SEM ($n = 4$ or 8) obtained from densitometric scans of data. $a_1 = P < .05$: compared with saline-saline group to test the effect of saline or caffeine injection. $b_1 = P < .05$: compared with saline-saline group to test the effect of drugs within saline treatment groups. $c_1 = P < .01$: compared with saline-caffeine group to test the effect of drugs within caffeine treatment groups. All statistical analyses were performed according to multiple comparisons with a control (Dunnett's t test). Saline-induced increases in *c-fos* were antagonized by diazepam, while caffeine-induced increases were selectively antagonized by NECA and increased by Ro 5-4864.

Uhde and Tancer 1989), repeated caffeine administration in panic disorder was not associated with the same degree of attenuation of caffeine's effects that was observed in normal volunteers. Thus, not only are there differences in sensitivity to caffeine's acute effects in panic patients and normal volunteers, but the adaptive changes to repeated challenge in these two groups may differ as well.

These findings are of interest in relation to the differential effects of repeated caffeine administration on different endpoints (hyperactivity vs. seizures) in different species. In the mouse, in which caffeine-induced *c-fos* induction involves only the striatum even after seizures, kindling-like increases in seizure sensitivity have been demonstrated (M. Clark et al., unpublished observations, 1990). In the rat, *c-fos* induction by subconvulsive doses of caffeine is limited to the striatum; however, with caffeine-induced seizures, *c-fos* inductions also include the dentate gyrus of the hippocampus, the olfactory bulb, and the cerebral cortex. In this species, high-dose caffeine fails to produce kindling-like seizure progression, and low-dose caffeine–induced hyperactivity shows a prominent pattern of tolerance. Thus, *c-fos* induction may help in elucidation of the anatomic substrates and mechanisms involved in tolerance and sensitization to repeated caffeine administration and, ultimately, to the substrate of caffeine-induced panic.

Cocaine-Induced *c-fos*: Limbic and Striatal Involvement

As noted above, the pattern of *c-fos* induction with cocaine appears to be a combination of that observed with amygdala-kindled seizures (largely limbic and cortical) and the pattern induced by caffeine (largely striatal and olfactory tubercle) (see Figure 4–11). The pattern of *c-fos* induction achieved by a single convulsive dose of cocaine was highly similar to that shown in the cocaine-kindled animal (Clark et al. 1992). A similar pattern of *c-fos* induction was also observed following acute lidocaine seizures, again with prominent involvement of the dentate gyrus of the hippocampus and a variety of cortical areas, and minor involvement of the striatum.

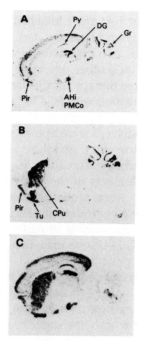

Figure 4–11. In situ hybridization of *c-fos* mRNA in sagittal sections of mouse brain. *(A)* Electroconvulsive seizure (ECS; see Figure 4–7 also). *(B)* Caffeine-induced seizure (see Figures 4–8 and 4–9 also). *(C)* Cocaine-induced seizure. Abbreviations: Py, pyramidal cells of the hippocampus; DG, dentate gyrus; Gr, granule cell layer of the cerebellum; AHi, amygdalohippocampal area; PMCo, posteromedial cortical amygdala nucleus; Pir, piriform cortex; CPu, caudate-putamen; Tu, olfactory tubercle. Note relative limbic distribution of *c-fos* induced by ECS *(A)*, striatal distribution with caffeine *(B)*, and a combination of both with cocaine *(C)*.

Pentylenetetrazole and FG 7142, An Inverse Benzodiazepine Agonist

Other panicogens have been shown by other investigators to induce *c-fos*. Morgan et al. (1987) reported *c-fos* induction by pentylenetetrazole in whole brain, and Dragunow and Robertson (1987) found that the increase in *c-fos* was selective to the dentate gyrus and the cingulate and piriform cortices. These findings are particularly noteworthy in light of the long history of anxiety and panic induced with pentylenetetrazole, particularly when this agent was originally given as a pharmacological convulsant for the treatment of affective and other psychotic disorders prior to the use of electroconvulsive therapy for this indication.

The finding of *c-fos* induction with FG 7142 is also noteworthy in terms of its mechanistic implications. FG 7142 is an inverse agonist acting on benzodiazepine receptors that exerts effects essentially opposite to those of the anxiolytic and anticonvulsant compounds diazepam and clonazepam. When FG 7142 was administered to several volunteers in the study of Dorow (1987), clear-cut panic reactions were produced that were reversible with intravenous doses of a benzodiazepine agonist. Thus, to the extent that the proto-oncogene *c-fos* provides a map of neural substrates activated by FG 7142, one may, in a preliminary fashion, begin to think of the potential neural substrates involved in different types of panic inductions. Comparisons and contrasts with caffeine and cocaine are particularly notable. The pattern induced by FG 7142 suggests hippocampal and cortical involvement, while that induced by caffeine suggests a primary role for the striatum.

Induction of *c-fos* by Yohimbine and Other Panicogens

The α_2 antagonist yohimbine has been reported to produce panic attacks in panic disorder patients but not in normal control subjects (Uhde 1990). Thus, given the preliminary suggestion of a potential for a differential responsivity to the panicogenic effects of yohimbine in panic patients compared with control subjects, we sought to explore the potential neural substrates activated by yohimbine with the in situ hybridization technique (J. Rosen, C. Cain, D. Fontana, unpublished observations). When yohimbine (10 mg/kg ip) produced seizures, notable increases in c-fos mRNA were induced in the dentate gyrus of the hippocampus as well as in widespread cortical areas (Figure 4–12). In contrast, when the same dose of yohimbine was administered and was not associated with a seizure, very little *c-fos* induction was observed. This was also the case with lower doses of yohimbine, including 7.5, 5.0, and 2.5 mg/kg, all of which did not produce seizures.

Thus, in contrast to the clear-cut dose-related *c-fos* inductions produced by the panicogen caffeine (see Figures 4–8 and 4–9), yohimbine appeared to produce these effects in an all-or-none fashion, with only minor effects achieved by subconvulsant doses of the drug.

Preliminary attempts to map *c-fos* inductions with other panicogens (by J. Rosen) led to similar results when subconvulsant doses of lactate (2.5 μmole/kg iv), *m*-chlorophenylpiperazine (10 mg/kg ip), isoproterenol (200 μg/kg sc), and cholecystokinin (100 μg/kg iv) were utilized. Therefore, it appears that either a) the in situ hybridization technique is not sensitive enough to pick up changes in *c-fos* induced by nonconvulsant doses of these substances, or b) *c-fos* induction emerges in a relatively all-or-none fashion following afterdischarges or seizures induced by

c-Fos mRNA

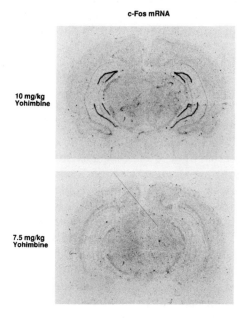

10 mg/kg
Yohimbine

7.5 mg/kg
Yohimbine

Figure 4–12. Pattern of *c-fos* induction achieved by convulsive doses (10 mg/kg ip) but not subconvulsive doses (7.5 mg/kg ip) of yohimbine, the α₂ antagonist that increases firing of the locus coeruleus and induces panic attacks in susceptible individuals.

these substances but not in lower doses or in a dose-related fashion, with the exception of caffeine.

Implications

To the extent that panic attacks are related to processes that are preconvulsant and/or near the convulsant threshold (achieved acutely or by a kindling-like mechanism), these data suggest that panic attacks might occur in a relatively all-or-none fashion with some chemical substances but not with others, such as caffeine, in which dose-related effects on anxiety may also be seen. These data are, in part, convergent with the dose-related changes in anxiety demonstrated by Uhde and associates (Uhde 1990; Uhde and Kellner 1987) in normal volunteers as well as dose-related changes in cortisol. These data may also explain the more widespread effects of caffeine and its avoidance by a much higher percentage of panic patients than in the normal population (Boulenger et al. 1984).

The chemical models described in this chapter show remarkable convergence regarding activation of the piriform cortex and dentate gyrus of the hippocampus in terms of *c-fos* induction. These data are noteworthy in relation to the emerging topographic mapping of panic anxiety disorder with cerebral blood flow and PET techniques in humans. The data of Reiman et al. (1986) suggest that there is a left-right asymmetry in the parahippocampal gyrus of patients with panic disorder who are prone to have panic attacks after administration of lactate, with increased blood flow in the right, compared with the left, parahippocampal gyrus. The prominent involvement of the hippocampus, which exerts negative control over cortisol secretion, could explain why most panicogens (with the exception of caffeine) are not associated with cortisol hypersecretion. Reiman et al. (1989a, 1989b) have followed up their initial blood flow studies with subsequent work which suggests that panic attacks or anticipatory anxiety (in normal volunteers) may produce increased blood flow in the temporal poles. Further studies are necessary to determine the importance of temporal lobe structures in panic anxiety disorders (Drevets et al. 1992), yet the convergence of the basic and clinical findings in this regard remains intriguing.

Possible Role of *c-fos* and Other Transcription Factors in the Long-Term Alterations in Responsivity in Panic Disorder Patients

The long-term consequences of *c-fos* induction are not definitively known. However, a preliminary picture is emerging to suggest that *c-fos* induction may be a first step in a cascade of a variety of longer-term adaptive changes in the organism (Berridge 1989; Crabtree 1989; Dragunow et al. 1989; Morgan and Curran 1989a, 1989b; Morgan et al. 1987). Thus, it is possible that with neurotransmission associated with receptor activation and second-messenger alterations, *c-fos* becomes induced as a third-messenger system. We briefly outline how this is likely to occur (Figure 4–13).

Once *c-fos* mRNA is induced, it leaves the nucleus to activate the ribosomes of the endoplasmic reticulum, where it is involved in the synthesis of Fos protein. Fos protein joins (via a leucine zipper) with another proto-oncogene product, Jun, to form a heterodimer. This Fos-Jun complex is more potent as a DNA binding substrate and transcription factor than homodimers of Fos or Jun alone. This Fos-Jun heterodimer is then translocated into the nucleus, where it binds to an AP1 site that is involved in subsequent alterations in gene transcription. As noted earlier, long-term alterations as a consequence of *c-fos* activation might include synthesis of new proteins, peptides, receptors, neurotransmitters, and structural proteins.

While we have focused on *c-fos* induction and its possible consequences in this discussion, it should be emphasized that *c-fos* is only one of many proto-oncogenes with a leucine-zipper motif, and this motif is only one of many (e.g., zinc-finger, copper-fist, etc.) that can be activated by extra- and intracellular events (Vinson et al. 1989). Thus, the timing and ratio of the mix of transcription factors appear capable of coding the complexity of intracellular events that vary on the basis of past experience and ongoing neural events. For example, Jun-B has different biological effects from, and is a negative regulator of, *c-jun* (Chiu et al. 1989). Moreover, it has recently been demonstrated that the transcription factor activities of the glucocorticoid receptor can inhibit those of *c-fos* or *c-jun* and vice versa (Lucibello et al. 1990), further indicating the possibility of "cross-talk" among classes of transcription factors that could be important to the precise timing of responses, based on associative processes and past experiences. In this fashion, the context of ongoing neural activity may be reflected by the presence, absence, or ratios of multiple transcription factors.

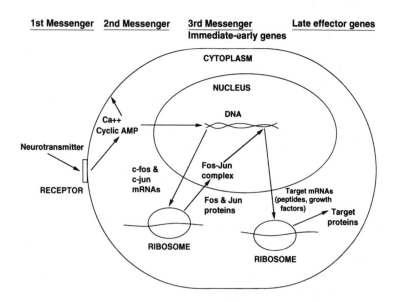

Figure 4–13. Schematic drawing of pathway for activation of *c-fos* and transcription of Fos-regulated proteins. Cells can be activated by release of various neurotransmitters, including glutamate and acetylcholine (first messengers). Following receptor activation, second messengers such as cAMP and Ca^{++} are formed or released and activate kinases that either phosphorylate cytosolic or membrane proteins, or induce transcription of *c-fos* and *c-jun* mRNA at DNA regulatory elements within the nucleus. The expressed mRNAs move into the cytoplasm, attach to ribosomes, and are translated into Fos and Jun proteins, respectively. The proteins (third messengers) then are translocated back into the nucleus to form the Fos-Jun complex that binds to the AP1 site on DNA to regulate transcription of other genes (possibly altering transmitters, synthetic enzymes, neuropeptides, growth factors, and membrane channels) in a transient or long-lasting fashion.

Sonnenberg et al. (1989) have hypothesized that following seizures *c-fos* is directly involved in the induction of the pre-pro-enkephalin gene, although this remains to be definitively demonstrated. Others have surmised that *c-fos* induction is, at least temporally, associated with a subsequent increase in somatostatin following amygdala-kindled seizures and a decrease in dynorphin mRNA in the same instance (Gall et al. 1990; Rosen et al. 1992; Shinoda et al. 1991). Smith et al. (1991) have also demonstrated that amygdala-kindled seizures transiently increase mRNA for CRH in the hippocampus. Thus, amygdala-kindled, seizure-induced *c-fos* mRNAs may be associated with transcription of mRNAs and their peptide products, with their associated long-lasting consequences for neural excitability.

One is now in a position to conceptualize how the experience of an acute panic attack might not only be associated with events at the level of neurotransmission but get encoded in a "memory-like fashion" by a series of downstream effects on longer-term neurotransmitter, receptor, peptide, and protein constituents that may convey long-lasting changes in responsivity for the organism. This schema becomes all the more attractive based on the notion that endogenous processes and stressors (Bullitt 1989; Ceccatelli et al. 1989; Daval et al 1989; Draisci and Iadarola 1989; Nakajima et al. 1989a, 1989b; Smith et al. 1991) are capable of inducing the proto-oncogene *c-fos* and thus are capable of entering the same hypothetical cascade. Obviously, much work remains to be done in order to directly demonstrate that similar types of processes initiated by *c-fos* induction following a seizure also occur following an exogenous stressor (or the endogenous changes associated with a panic attack). Nonetheless, preliminary data demonstrating stress-induced and CRH-induced increases in *c-fos* clearly raise the possibility that this type of putative mechanism for conveying long-lasting changes in the organism is more than a theoretical possibility (Figure 4–14).

Bolstering this argument is the work of Steven Rose, who has demonstrated various elements in this cascade following a single trial of conditioned avoidance learning in the neonatal chick. In his model, 1-day-old chicks are observed to readily peck at a shiny bright metal object and continue to do this if a water reward emanates from the metal object. If the water is substituted with a bitter-tasting substance, the chicks learn, on the basis of a single trial, to avoid this shiny metal object in a relatively permanent fashion. Rose and colleagues (Rose 1991; Patterson et al. 1990) have demonstrated that regionally specific inductions of *c-fos* emerge following this one-trial avoidance learning in the chick and are followed by a variety of downstream consequences in other neurochemical systems. These neurochemical changes,

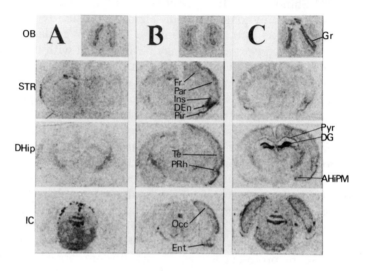

Figure 4–14. Effect of intracerebroventricular CRF on *c-fos* induction. In situ hybridization of *c-fos* mRNA in coronal sections of rat brain at the levels of olfactory bulb (OB), striatum (STR), dorsal hippocampus (DHip), and inferior colliculus (IC). *(A)* Rat injected with sterile water (vehicle). *(B)* Rat injected with corticotropin-releasing hormone (CRH) but not having a seizure. Note unilateral increase in *c-fos* mRNA in the dorsal endopiriform nucleus (DEn) and in the piriform (Pir), insular (Ins), frontal (Fr), parietal (Par), temporal (Te), perirhinal (PRh), occipital (Occ), and entorhinal (Ent) cortices. *(C)* Rat injected with CRH and having seizures. Note bilateral cortical and hippocampal involvement with the seizure state. All three rats were sacrificed at approximately 3 hours after the injection (icv). Other abbreviations: Gr, granular layer of the olfactory bulb; DG, dentate gyrus; Pyr, pyramidal cell layer of the hippocampus; AHiPM, posteromedial amygdalo-hippocampal area.

based on experience and learning, are also associated with microanatomic changes at the level of synaptic densities, spine formation, and synapse formation.

It is also of interest that the macroanatomy of this process seems to migrate with time, initially residing in the left dorsal part of the brain, transferring to the right side, moving ventrally, and then back to the ventral left portion of the brain, as assessed by the effects of lesions on the ability to retain this memory. Thus, in a situation of one-trial learning (which presumably has very minor arousing and signaling consequences to the organism, in contrast to a panic attack), not only has *c-fos* induction been shown to occur as part of a cascade of neurobiological effects, but it appears to be intimately involved in processes of learning and memory that have their microstructural and migrating macro-neuroanatomic residues for the putative memory trace of this experience.

Recent work from the laboratory of Julius Axelrod is also indirectly supportive of the notion that *fos* and *jun* are intimately involved in altered cellular reactivity based on prior experience or exposure (Fagarasan et al. 1990). β-Endorphin secretion is measured in cultured AtT-20 cells stimulated by interleukin-1. Upon a second challenge with interleukin-1, an increased secretion of β-endorphin is observed. Treating the cells with the antisense (i.e., a selective inhibitor) of either *c-fos* or *c-jun* alone was insufficient to block the increased secretion of β-endorphin following interleukin-1 rechallenge. However, introduction of antisense RNA to both substances together did block this process, suggesting that the presence of either *fos* or *jun* alone was sufficient to confer the enhanced responsivity of these cells, but that blockade of both substances (perhaps at the level of the effects of the heterodimer on the AP1 binding site) inhibited the sensitized responses.

The induction of another immediate-early gene, *zif/268*, is closely linked to activation of NMDA receptors in long-term potentiation, which is a model for memory in the hippocampal slice (Cole et al. 1989). Other animal systems may be useful in documenting the role of biochemical and structural changes in learning and memory paradigms, particularly related to the development of anxiety (Glanzman et al. 1990; Kandel 1983). Nelson et al. (1990), working with Hermissenda, suggest that a variety of mRNAs are induced with associative learning, but not when the same stimuli are presented in an unpaired fashion, in which case no learning takes place.

Taken together, these data suggest the possibility that initial spontaneous or biochemically induced panic attacks may occur in such fashion as not only to acutely perturb the organism but also to leave a residual or "memory" trace behind that could alter subsequent responsivity. These putative plastic changes could lead to either increases or decreases in the likelihood of recurrent panic attacks, as well as form the substrate for conditioned associations to the situation surrounding the panic attack, leading to the development of agoraphobia (Uhde et al. 1985).

IMPLICATIONS FOR PHARMACOTHERAPEUTICS AND CONTINGENT TOLERANCE

Pharmacology as a Function of Stage of Illness?

We have previously hinted at the potential implications of the kindling model for pharmacotherapeutics. Pharmacological interventions effective in the initial developing phase of kindling may not be effective in the completed phase or in the spontaneous phase, and vice versa (Table 4–1). These powerful pharmacological dissociations in kindling have now been well replicated (Post et al. 1991). In addition, they are also clearly apparent in other models such as long-term potentiation, in which substances that can block the development of long-term potentiation are different from those that interfere with its maintenance or expression. In a parallel fashion, it is possible that pharmacological interventions in the course of the evolution of panic disorders may differ as a function of stage of development. This could be tested directly in the model of cocaine-induced panic attack evolution, in which carbamazepine, in particular, would be predicted to be effective in preventing the evolution of cocaine-related panic attacks. High-potency anticonvulsant benzodiazepines should also block the development and completed phases, but the efficacy of these substances in the later spontaneous phase of the disorder remains to be systematically tested.

Thus, it is possible that the psychopharmacology of panic disorder, specifically in relation to cocaine-induced panic attacks and possibly in the spontaneous variety as well, could differ as a function of stage of evolution. While the data supporting this proposition are at least convergent with the existing literature for the psychopharmacology of the affective disorders (Post et al. 1986a), there is relatively less information available for panic disorder. The present formulation is presented to raise this possibility and stimulate the conduct of clinical trials that might prove or disprove this hypothesis.

Contingent Tolerance and Its Reversal

A final preclinical model may have important implications for the pharmacotherapeutics of panic anxiety disorders. In attempting to suppress completed amygdala-kindled seizures with the anticonvulsant carbamazepine, Weiss and Post (1991a, 1991b, in press) observed inconsistent effects of this agent with repeated once-daily administration. When studies were performed in a systematic fashion, it became apparent that repeated once-daily administration of carbamazepine (15 mg/kg ip), which was initially effective in inhibiting completed amygdala-kindled seizures (see Figure 4–15, day 23), over a period of 4 to 7 days, became ineffective. This kind of tolerance to anticonvulsants such as carbamazepine or diazepam on amygdala-kindled seizures was contingent on the presence of the drug at the time of the kindled stimulation and did not emerge when the animals were kindled and then given the drug immediately after the kindled stimulation.

Thus, the temporal pairing of drug and seizure appeared critical to the induction of tolerance. Once tolerance to the anticonvulsant effects of carbamazepine was induced, it could be reversed by either a period of kindling the animal with no medication at all or giving the animal kindled seizures with the drug administered after the occurrence of the seizure (see Figure 4–15, days 49–55). Tolerance remained if the animals were left without kindling stimulation or drug treatment, or if they were treated with carbamazepine alone. These data suggest that it is the specific occurrence of a seizure in the absence of drug that

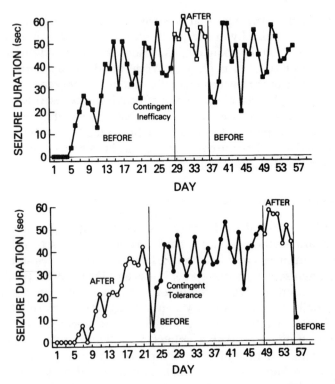

Figure 4–15. Contingent inefficacy and tolerance to carbamazepine reversal with treatment *after* kindled seizures. The group mean seizure duration is illustrated for animals receiving carbamazepine (15 mg/kg ip) before *(top)* or after *(bottom)* amygdala kindling stimulation on a once-daily basis. The two groups are plotted separately to facilitate comparison over a longer period of time. *Top:* The group receiving carbamazepine before kindled seizures did not respond to treatment at a time when the group receiving carbamazepine after seizures was responsive (contingent inefficacy). (For comparison see days 23–25 (bottom); also see Weiss and Post 1991a for details). *Bottom:* The group receiving carbamazepine after kindled seizures showed a good anticonvulsant response to carbamazepine treatment before kindled seizures (days 23–25) ($P < .01$) but became tolerant to this effect (days 26–48). A subsequent period of 7 days of kindled seizures *followed* by drug (i.e., carbamazepine was given *after* stimulation [days 49-55]) reinstated the anticonvulsant efficacy of carbamazepine (day 56) ($P < .05$).

led to the reversal of the contingent tolerance.

In this paradigm, it is apparent that differential consequences for efficacy of the drug are solely dependent on the temporal order (pairing) of drug and seizure induction. If the drug is administered prior to the seizure induction, tolerance will develop; if it is administered after the seizure has occurred, not only does tolerance not occur, but this unpairing is sufficient to renew clinical efficacy (Weiss and Post 1991a, 1991b). These data and others are highly suggestive that pharmacokinetic factors are not important to this model of contingent tolerance.

Recent clinical data are consistent with this model. Doyle and associates (1990) have observed better responsivity by epileptic patients to their anticonvulsants following a period of medication-free evaluation than was initially observed. We have speculated elsewhere that this development of contingent tolerance may also be pertinent to the development of loss of efficacy in patients with trigeminal neuralgia and recurrent affective disorders (Pazzaglia and Post, in press; Post et al. 1990). In a parallel fashion, we would wonder whether the contingent tolerance phenomenon might not also be worthy of consideration when an antipanic treatment that was initially effective begins to show a pattern of tolerance development. Although this is not a widely occurring phenomenon in the literature, it may be a relevant variable in at least a subgroup of patients who develop refractoriness to an initially effective antipanic drug treatment.

In these instances of tolerance development, one might question whether a period of time off medications might be sufficient to renew clinical antipanic efficacy in a fashion parallel to that observed in the preclinical tolerance model. Obviously, another option in the face of the emerging tolerance is to switch to another drug with a different mechanism of action. For example, in the preclinical model, Weiss and Post (1991a) have observed that once the animals have become tolerant to the anticonvulsant effects of carbamazepine, they are cross-tolerant to PK 11195, which is active at peripheral-type benzodiazepine receptors in a fashion similar to that of carbamazepine (Figure 4–16). In contrast, animals tolerant to the anticonvulsant effects of carbamazepine were still responsive to the anticonvulsant effects of diazepam, an agent that is active at central-type benzodiazepine receptors (Weiss et al. 1985). Therefore, in the face of emerging loss of efficacy to antipanic pharmacotherapy based on a contingent tolerance paradigm, one might consider either 1) a period of time off the medication and then renewed challenge with that same drug, or 2) treatment with a novel agent with a different mechanism of action.

The differential role of benzodiazepine receptors in different types of tolerance development is elegantly demonstrated in the study by Mana and Pinel (1990). They documented that noncontingent tolerance development to the central-type benzodiazepine ligand diazepam was reversed by the specific antagonist RO 15-1788, whereas contingent tolerance was not. Thus, contingent tolerance development to a variety of agents may follow different biochemical pathways from those associated with more

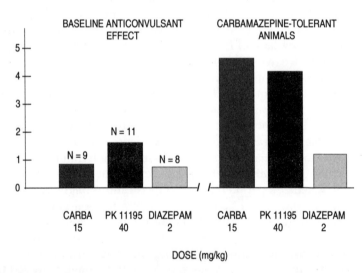

Figure 4–16. Cross-tolerance between carbamazepine and peripheral-type, but not central-type, benzodiazepine ligands. The group mean seizure stage is plotted for animals on the first day of anticonvulsant administration *(left half)* and following the induction of tolerance to carbamazepine *(right half)* when animals experienced full-blown stage-4/stage-5 seizures despite drug pretreatment. Cross-tolerance to the peripheral-type benzodiazepine ligand PK 11195 is observed but not to the central-type benzodiazepine ligand diazepam.

traditional tolerance development based on chronic exposure to a drug. In this regard, Pinel and associates have demonstrated contingent tolerance to the anticonvulsant effects of benzodiazepines and alcohol (Pinel and Mana 1986; Mana and Pinel 1990). Our new findings for carbamazepine suggest that even with a drug that is not usually associated with tolerance development (as are alcohol and benzodiazepines), contingent alterations in seizure threshold (Weiss et al. 1991) and the loss of pharmacoresponsivity can be clearly demonstrated, at least in a seizure model.

Obviously, much work is required in order to explore the possible clinical relevance and ramifications of these preclinical observations. We would highlight the possible utility of considering the efficacy of pharmacotherapeutic drugs in light of contingent manipulations that can make a drug effective or ineffective, depending on its temporal associations with the condition to be treated. The paroxysmal nature of panic attacks would suggest that contingent tolerance could be engendered as has been demonstrated in seizure disorders and is now suggested with paroxysmal pain syndromes such as trigeminal neuralgia. In addition to these potential clinical implications, we would also suggest that the contingent tolerance paradigm is a robust and novel procedure that can be used to explicate molecular mechanisms involved in the "learned" or "contingent" nature of pharmacoresponsivity. These mechanisms may have important implications in their own right.

We have elaborated a series of preclinical models that may have interesting implications for the evolution and treatment of patients with panic anxiety disorder. We have tried to raise these issues in a preliminary and speculative note with the hope of engendering further studies of these phenomena and their potential relevance to the clinical disorders of paroxysmal anxiety.

References

Adamec R: Behavioral and epileptic determinants of predatory attack behavior in the cat. Can J Neurol Sci 2:457–466, 1975

Alldredge BK, Lowenstein DH, Simon RP: Seizures associated with recreational drug abuse. Neurology 39:1037–1039, 1989

Angrist BM, Gershon S: The phenomenology of experimentally induced amphetamine psychosis—preliminary observations. Biol Psychiatry 2:95–107, 1970

Antelman SM: Stressor-induced sensitization to subsequent stress: implications for the development and treatment of clinical disorders, in Sensitization in the Nervous System. Edited by Kalivas PW, Barnes CD. Caldwell, NJ, Telford Press, 1988, pp 227–254

Antelman SM, Eichler AJ, Black CA, et al: Interchangeability of stress and amphetamine in sensitization. Science 207:329–331, 1980

Anthony JC, Tien AY, Petronis KR: Epidemiologic evidence on cocaine use and panic attacks. Am J Epidemiol 129:543–549, 1989

Arenander AT, de Vellis J, Herschman HR: Induction of c-fos and TIS genes in cultured rat astrocytes by neurotransmitters. J Neurosci Res 24:107–114, 1989

Aronson TA, Craig TJ: Cocaine precipitation of panic disorder. Am J Psychiatry 143:643–645, 1986

Baxter LR Jr, Schwartz JM, Phelps ME, et al: Localization of neurochemical effects of cocaine and other stimulants in the human brain. J Clin Psychiatry 49:23–26, 1988

Berridge MJ: The Albert Lasker Medical Awards: inositol trisphosphate, calcium, lithium, and cell signaling. JAMA 262:1834–1841, 1989

Boulenger J-P, Uhde TW: Caffeine consumption and anxiety: preliminary results of a survey comparing patients with anxiety disorders and normal controls. Psychopharmacol Bull 18:53–57, 1982

Boulenger J-P, Uhde TW, Wolff EA, et al: Increased sensitivity to caffeine in patients with panic disorders: preliminary evidence. Arch Gen Psychiatry 41:1067–1071, 1984

Bravo R, Neuberg M, Burkhardt J, et al: Involvement of common and cell type–specific pathways in c-fos gene control: stable induction by cAMP in macrophages. Cell 48:251–260, 1987

Bullitt E: Induction of c-fos–like protein within the lumbar spinal cord and thalamus of the rat following peripheral stimulation. Brain Res 493:391–397, 1989

Burchfiel JL, Applegate CD, Samoriski GM: Evidence for piriform cortex as a critical substrate for the stepwise progression of kindling. Epilepsia 31:632, 1990

Cain DP, Corcoran ME: Intracerebral beta-endorphin, met-enkephalin and morphine: kindling of seizures and handling-induced potentiation of epileptiform effects. Life Sci 34:2535–2542, 1984

Calogero AE, Kling MA, Bernardini R, et al: Cocaine stimulates rat hypothalamic corticotropin-releasing hormone secretion in vitro. Clin Research 36:361, 1988

Ceccatelli S, Villar MJ, Goldstein M, et al: Expression of c-fos immuno-reactivity in transmitter-characterized neurons after stress. Proc Natl Acad Sci U S A 86:9569–9573, 1989

Charney DS, Heninger GR: Noradrenergic function and the mechanism of action of antianxiety treatment, I: the effect of long-term alpra-zolam treatment. Arch Gen Psychiatry 42:458–467, 1985

Childress AR, McLellan AT, Ehrman RN, et al: Extinction of conditioned responses in abstinent cocaine or opioid users. NIDA Res Monogr 76:189–195, 1987

Childress A, Ehrman R, McLellan AT, et al: Conditioned craving and arousal in cocaine addiction: a preliminary report. NIDA Res Monogr 81:74–80, 1988

Chiu R, Angel P, Karin M: Jun-B differs in its biological properties from, and is a negative regulator of, c-Jun. Cell 59:979–986, 1989

Clark M, Post RM, Weiss SRB, et al: Regional expression of c-fos mRNA in rat brain during the evolution of amygdala kindled seizures. Brain Res Mol Brain Res 11:55–64, 1991a

Clark M, Weiss SRB, Post RM: Expression of c-fos mRNA in rat brain after intracerebroventricular administration of corticotropin-releas-ing hormone. Neurosci Lett 132:235–238, 1991b

Clark M, Post RM, Weiss SRB, et al: Expression of c–fos mRNA in acute and kindled cocaine seizures in rats. Brain Res 582:101–106, 1992

Cole AJ, Saffen DW, Baraban JM, et al: Rapid increase of an immediate-early gene messenger RNA in hippocampal neurons by synaptic NMDA receptor activation. Nature 340:474–476, 1989

Connell PH, Akkerhuis GW: Amphetamine Psychosis (Maudsley Monogr No 5). New York, Oxford University Press, 1958

Coppola R, Salb J, Chassey J: Topographic analysis of epileptiform dis-charges. Abstract of paper presented at the 15th Epilepsy Interna-tional Symposium, Washington, DC, September 1983

Crabtree GR: Contingent genetic regulatory events in T lymphocyte activation. Science 243:355–361, 1989

Daval JL, Nakajima T, Gleiter CH, et al: Mouse brain c-fos mRNA distri-bution following a single electroconvulsive shock. J Neurochem 52:1954–1957, 1989

De Jong RH, Walts LF: Lidocaine-induced psychomotor seizures in man. Acta Anaesthesiol Scand Suppl 23:598–604, 1966

Dhuna A, Pascual-Leone A: New onset seizures after first-time cocaine abuse. Epilepsia 31:605, 1990

Dorow R: FG 7142 and its anxiety-inducing effects in humans. Br J Clin Pharmacol 23:781–782, 1987

Downs AW, Eddy NB: The effect of repeated doses of cocaine on the dog. J Pharmacol Exp Ther 46:195, 1932a

Downs AW, Eddy NB: The effect of repeated doses of cocaine on the rat. J Pharmacol Exp Ther 46:199–200, 1932b

Doyle WK, Devinsky O, Perrine K, et al: Decreased frequency of seizures after antiepileptic drug holiday in medically refractory epilepsy (abstract). Epilepsia 31:640, 1990

Dragunow M, Faull RL: Rolipram induces c-fos protein–like immunoreactivity in ependymal and glial-like cells in adult rat brain. Brain Res 501:382–388, 1989

Dragunow M, Robertson HA: Generalized seizures induce c-fos protein(s) in mammalian neurons. Neurosci Lett 82:157–161, 1987

Dragunow M, Abraham WC, Goulding M, et al: Long-term potentiation and the induction of c-fos mRNA and proteins in the dentate gyrus of unanesthetized rats. Neurosci Lett 101:274–280, 1989

Draisci G, Iadarola MJ: Temporal analysis of increases in c-fos, preprodynorphin and preproenkephalin mRNAs in rat spinal cord. Brain Res Mol Brain Res 6:31–37, 1989

Drevets WC, Videen TO, MacLeod AK, et al: PET images of blood flow changes during anxiety: correction. Science 256:1696, 1992

Ehlers CL, Henriksen SJ, Wang M, et al: Corticotropin-releasing factor produces increases in brain excitability and convulsive seizures in rats. Brain Res 278:332–336, 1983

Ellinwood EH: Amphetamine psychosis: individuals, settings, and sequences, in Current Concepts in Amphetamine Abuse (NIMH Publication HSM 72-9085). Washington, DC, U.S. Government Printing Office, 1972, pp 143–157

Ellinwood EH, Kilbey MM, Castellani S, et al: Amygdala hyperspindling and seizures induced by cocaine, in Advances in Behavioral Biology, Vol 21: Cocaine and Other Stimulants. Edited by Ellinwood EH, Kilbey MM. New York, Plenum, 1977, pp 303–326

Emmett-Oglesby MW, Wurst M, Lal H: Discriminative stimulus properties of a small dose of cocaine. Neuropharmacology 22:97–101, 1983

Fagarasan MO, Aiello F, Muegge K, et al: Interleukin 1 induces beta-endorphin secretion via Fos and Jun in AtT-20 pituitary cells. Proc Natl Acad Sci U S A 87:7871–7874, 1990

Fischman MW, Schuster CR, Resnekov L, et al: Cardiovascular and subjective effects of intravenous cocaine administration in humans. Arch Gen Psychiatry 33:983–989, 1976

Fischman MW, Schuster CR, Hatano Y: A comparison of the subjective and cardiovascular effects of cocaine and lidocaine in humans. Pharmacol Biochem Behav 18:123–127, 1983a

Fischman MW, Schuster CR, Rajfer S: A comparison of the subjective and cardiovascular effects of cocaine and procaine in humans. Pharmacol Biochem Behav 18:711–716, 1983b

Gall C, Lauterborn J, Isackson P, et al: Seizures, neuropeptide regulation, and mRNA expression in the hippocampus. Prog Brain Res 83:371–390, 1990

Gawin FH, Ellinwood EH Jr: Cocaine and other stimulants: actions, abuse, and treatment. N Engl J Med 318:1173–1182, 1988

Gawin FH, Ellinwood EH Jr: Cocaine dependence. Annu Rev Med 40:149–161, 1989

Gawin FH, Kleber H: Issues in cocaine abuse treatment research, in Cocaine: Clinical and Biobehavioral Aspects. Edited by Fisher S, Raskin A, Uhlenhuth EH. New York, Oxford University Press, 1987, pp 174–192

Glanzman DL, Kandel ER, Schacher S: Target-dependent structural changes accompanying long-term synaptic facilitation in Aplysia neurons. Science 249:799–802, 1990

Goddard GV, McIntyre DC, Leech CK: A permanent change in brain function resulting from daily electrical stimulation. Exp Neurol 25:295–330, 1969

Goeders NE, Smith JE: Cortical dopaminergic involvement in cocaine reinforcement. Science 221:773–775, 1983

Goodman LS, Gilman A: The Pharmacological Basis of Therapeutics. New York, Macmillan, 1970

Gubits RM, Smith TM, Fairhurst JL, et al: Adrenergic receptors mediate changes in c-fos mRNA levels in brain. Brain Res Mol Brain Res 6:39–45, 1989

Halgren E, Walter RD, Cherlow DG, et al: Mental phenomena evoked by electrical stimulation of the human hippocampal formation and amygdala. Brain 101:83–117, 1978

Hunt SP, Pini A, Evan G: Induction of c-fos–like protein in spinal cord neurons following sensory stimulation. Nature 328:632–634, 1987

Kandel ER: From metapsychology to molecular biology: explorations into the nature of anxiety. Am J Psychiatry 140:1277–1293, 1983

Kellner CH, Post RM, Putnam F, et al: Intravenous procaine as a probe of limbic system activity in psychiatric patients and normal controls. Biol Psychiatry 22:1107–1126, 1987

Kelly PH, Iversen SD: Selective 60HDA-induced destruction of mesolimbic dopamine neurons: abolition of psychostimulant-induced locomotor activity in rats. Eur J Pharmacol 40:45–56, 1976

Lathers CM, Tyau LSY, Spino MM, et al: Cocaine-induced seizures, arrhythmias and sudden death. J Clin Pharmacol 28:584–593, 1988

Louie AK, Lannon RA, Ketter TA: Treatment of cocaine-induced panic disorder. Am J Psychiatry 146:40–44, 1989

Lucibello FC, Slater EP, Jooss KU, et al: Mutual transrepression of Fos and the glucocorticoid receptor: involvement of a functional domain in Fos which is absent in FosB. EMBO J 9:2827–2834, 1990

Mana MJ, Pinel JPJ: RO 15-1788 reverses pharmacologic tolerance, but not contingent tolerance, to diazepam's anticonvulsant effect. Abstracts of the Society for Neuroscience, No 16, 1990

Merriam AE, Medalia A, Levine B: Partial complex status epilepticus associated with cocaine abuse. Biol Psychiatry 23:515–518, 1988

Meyendorff E, Lerer B, Moore NC, et al: Methylphenidate infusion in euthymic bipolars: effect of carbamazepine pretreatment. Psychiatry Res 16:303, 1985

Morgan JI, Curran T: Role of ion flux in the control of c-fos expression. Nature 322:552–555, 1986

Morgan JI, Curran T: Calcium as a modulator of the immediate-early gene cascade in neurons. Cell Calcium 9:303–311, 1988

Morgan JI, Curran T: Calcium and proto-oncogene involvement in the immediate-early response in the nervous system. Ann N Y Acad Sci 568:283–290, 1989a

Morgan JI, Curran T: Stimulus-transcription coupling in neurons: role of cellular immediate-early genes. Trends Neurosci 12:459–462, 1989b

Morgan JI, Cohen DR, Hempstead JL, et al: Mapping patterns of c-fos expression in the central nervous system after seizure. Science 237:192–197, 1987

Myers JA, Earnest MP: Generalized seizures and cocaine abuse. Neurology 34:675–676, 1984

Nakajima T, Daval JL, Gleiter CH, et al: c-fos mRNA expression following electrical-induced seizure and acute nociceptive stress in mouse brain. Epilepsy Res 4:156–159, 1989a

Nakajima T, Daval JL, Morgan PF, et al: Adenosinergic modulation of caffeine-induced c-fos mRNA expression in mouse brain. Brain Res 501:307–314, 1989b

Nakajima T, Post RM, Weiss SRB, et al: Perspectives on the mechanism of action of electroconvulsive therapy: anticonvulsant, dopaminergic, and c-fos oncogene effects. Convulsive Therapy 5:274–295, 1989c

Nelson TJ, Collin C, Alkon DL: Isolation of a G protein that is modified by learning and reduces potassium currents in hermissenda. Science 247:1479–1483, 1990

Ogunyemi AO, Locke GE, Kramer LD, et al: Complex partial status epilepticus provoked by "crack" cocaine. Ann Neurol 26:785–786, 1989

Patterson TA, Gilbert DB, Rose SP: Pre- and post-training lesions of the intermediate medial hyperstriatum ventrale and passive avoidance learning in the chick. Exp Brain Res 80:189–195, 1990

Pazzaglia PJ, Post RM: Contingent tolerance and re-response to carbamazepine: a case study in a patient with trigeminal neuralgia and bipolar disorder. J Neuropsychiatry Clin Neurosci (in press)

Peterson SL, Albertson TE: Neurotransmitter and neuromodulator function in the kindled seizure and state. Prog Neurobiol 19:237–270, 1982

Pinel JPJ: Kindling-induced experimental epilepsy in rats: cortical stimulation. Exp Neurol 72:559–569, 1981

Pinel JPJ, Mana MJ: Kindled seizures and drug tolerance, in Kindling 3. Edited by Wada JA. New York, Raven, 1986, pp 393–407

Pitts DK, Marwah J: Electrophysiological actions of cocaine on noradrenergic neurons in rat locus coeruleus. J Pharmacol Exp Ther 240:345–351, 1987a

Pitts DK, Marwah J: Reciprocal pre- and post-synaptic actions of cocaine at a central noradrenergic synapse. Exp Neurol 98:518–528, 1987b

Post RM, Contel NR: Human and animal studies of cocaine: implications for development of behavioral pathology, in Stimulants: Neurochemical, Behavioral, and Clinical Perspective. Edited by Creese I. New York, Raven, 1983, pp 169–203

Post RM, Kopanda RT, Lee A: Progressive behavioral changes during chronic lidocaine administration: relationship to kindling. Life Sci 17:943–950, 1975

Post RM, Kopanda RT, Black KE: Progressive effects of cocaine on behavior and central amine metabolism in rhesus monkeys: relationship to kindling and psychosis. Biol Psychiatry 11:403–419, 1976

Post RM, Lockfeld A, Squillace KM, et al: Drug-environment interaction: context dependency of cocaine-induced behavioral sensitization. Life Sci 28:755–760, 1981

Post RM, Kennedy C, Shinohara M, et al: Metabolic and behavioral consequences of lidocaine-kindled seizures. Brain Res 324:295–303, 1984a

Post RM, Rubinow DR, Ballenger JC: Conditioning, sensitization, and kindling: implications for the course of affective illness, in Neurobiology of Mood Disorders. Edited by Post RM, Ballenger JC. Baltimore, MD, Williams & Wilkins, 1984b, pp 432–466

Post RM, Weiss SRB, Pert A: Differential effects of carbamazepine and lithium on sensitization and kindling. Prog Neuropsychopharmacol Biol Psychiatry 8:425–434, 1984c

Post RM, Rubinow DR, Ballenger JC: Conditioning and sensitization in the longitudinal course of affective illness. Br J Psychiatry 149:191–201, 1986a

Post RM, Uhde TW, Joffe RT, et al: Psychiatric manifestations and implications of seizure disorders, in Medical Mimics of Psychiatric Disorders. Edited by Extein I, Gold M. Washington, DC, American Psychiatric Press, 1986b, pp 35–91

Post RM, Weiss SRB, Pert A: The role of context and conditioning in behavioral sensitization to cocaine. Abstracts of the American College of Neuropsychopharmacology, no 63, 1986c

Post RM, Weiss SRB, Szele F, et al: Differential anticonvulsant effects of carbamazepine as a function of stage and type of kindling, in Abstracts of the Society for Neuroscience, no 374.1, 1986d, p 1375

Post RM, Weiss SRB, Pert A, et al: Chronic cocaine administration: sensitization and kindling effects, in Cocaine: Clinical and Biobehavioral Aspects. Edited by Raskin A, Fisher S. New York, Oxford University Press, 1987a, pp 109–173

Post RM, Weiss SRB, Pert A: The role of context in conditioning and behavioral sensitization to cocaine. Psychopharmacol Bull 23:425–429, 1987b

Post RM, Weiss SRB, Pert A: Cocaine-induced behavioral sensitization and kindling: implications for the emergence of psychopathology and seizures, in Mesocorticolimbic Dopamine System. Edited by Kalivas PW, Nemeroff CB. New York, New York Academy of Science, 1988, pp 292–308

Post RM, Weiss SRB, Clark M, et al: Amygdala versus local anesthetic kindling: differential anatomy, pharmacology, and clinical implications, in Kindling IV. Edited by Wada J. New York, Plenum, 1990, pp 357–369

Post RM, Weiss SRB, Clark M: Evolving anatomy and pharmacology of kindling. Abstracts of paper presented at the World Congress of Biological Psychiatry, Florence, Italy, June 1991

Racine RJ: Modification of seizure activity by electrical stimulation, II: motor seizure. Electroencephalogr Clin Neurophysiol 32:281–294, 1972

Redmond DE Jr, Huang YH: Current concepts, II. new evidence for a locus coeruleus–norepinephrine connection with anxiety. Life Sci 25:2149–2162, 1979

Reiman EM, Raichle ME, Robins E, et al: The application of positron emission tomography to the study of panic disorder. Am J Psychiatry 143:469–477, 1986

Reiman EM, Fusselman MJ, Fox PT, et al: Neuroanatomical correlates of anticipatory anxiety. Science 243:1071–1074, 1989a

Reiman EM, Raichle ME, Robins E, et al: Neuroanatomical correlates of a lactate-induced anxiety attack. Arch Gen Psychiatry 46:493–500, 1989b

Ritz MC, Lamb RJ, Goldberg SR, et al: Cocaine receptors on dopamine transporters are related to self-administration of cocaine. Science 237:1219–1223, 1987

Rivier C, Vale W: Cocaine stimulates adrenocorticotropin (ACTH) secretion through a corticotropin-releasing factor (CRF)–mediated mechanism. Brain Res 422:403–406, 1987

Roberts DCS, Koob GF, Klanoff P, et al: Extinction and recovery of cocaine self-administration following 6-hydroxydopamine lesions of the nucleus accumbens. Pharmacol Biochem Behav 12:781–787, 1980

Rose SP: How chicks make memories: the cellular cascade from c-fos to dendritic remodelling. Trends Neurosci 14:390–397, 1991

Rosen JB, Cain CJ, Weiss SRB, et al: Alterations in mRNA of enkephalin, dynorphin, and thyrotropin releasing hormone during amygdala kindling: an in situ hybridization study. Brain Res Mol Brain Res (in press)

Saravay SM, Marie J, Steinberg MD, et al: "Doom anxiety" and delirium in lidocaine toxicity. Am J Psychiatry 144:159–163, 1987

Shibanuma M, Kuroki T, Nose K: Inhibition of proto-oncogene c-fos transcription by inhibitors of protein kinase C and ion transport. Eur J Biochem 164:15–19, 1987

Shinoda H, Nadi NS, Schwartz JP: Alteration in somatostatin and proenkephalin mRNA in response to a single amygdaloid stimulation versus kindling. Brain Res Mol Brain Res 11:221–226, 1991

Smith M, Weiss SRB, Abedin T, et al: Effects of amygdala-kindling and electroconvulsive seizures on the expression of corticotropin releasing hormone (CRH) mRNA in the rat brain. Molecular and Cellular Neurosciences 2:103–116, 1991

Sonnenberg JL, Rauscher FJ III, Morgan JI, et al: Regulation of proenkephalin by Fos and Jun. Science 246:1622–1625, 1989

Stevens JR, Mark VH, Ervin F, et al: Deep temporal stimulation in man. Arch Neurol 21:157–167, 1969

Tramontano D, Chin WW, Moses AC, et al: Thyrotropin and dibutyryl cyclic AMP increase levels of c-myc and c-fos mRNAs in cultured rat thyroid cells. J Biol Chem 261:3919–3922, 1986

Uhde TW: Caffeine provocation of panic: a focus on biological mechanisms, in Neurobiology of Panic Disorder. Edited by Ballenger JC. New York, A R Liss, 1990, pp 365–376

Uhde TW, Kellner CH: Cerebral ventricular size in panic disorder. J Affective Disord 12:175–178, 1987

Uhde TW, Tancer ME: Chemical models of panic: a review and critique, in Psychopharmacology of Anxiety. Edited by Tyrer P. London, Oxford University Press, 1989, pp 109–131

Uhde TW, Boulenger JP, Post RM, et al: Fear and anxiety: relationship to noradrenergic function. Psychopathology 17:8–23, 1984

Uhde TW, Boulenger J-P, Roy-Byrne PP, et al: Longitudinal course of panic disorder: clinical and biological considerations. Prog Neuropsychopharmacol Biol Psychiatry 9:39–51, 1985

Uhde TW, Tancer ME, Gurguis GNM: Chemical models of anxiety: evidence for diagnostic and neurotransmitter specificity. International Review of Psychiatry 2:367–384, 1990

Vinson CR, Sigler PB, McKnight SL: Scissors-grip model for DNA recognition by a family of leucine zipper proteins. Science 246:911–916, 1989

Wada JA, Sato M, Corcoran ME: Persistent seizure susceptibility and recurrent spontaneous seizures in kindled cats. Epilepsia 15:465–478, 1974

Washton AM, Gold MS: Chronic cocaine abuse: evidence for adverse effects on health and functioning. Psychiatric Annals 14:733–743, 1984

Washton AM, Gold MS: Recent trends in cocaine abuse: a view from the National Hotline, "800-COCAINE." Adv Alcohol Subst Abuse 6:31–47, 1986

Washton AM, Tatarsky A: Adverse effects of cocaine abuse. NIDA Res Monogr 49:247–254, 1984

Weiss SRB, Post RM: Contingent tolerance to carbamazepine: a peripheral-type benzodiazepine mechanism. Eur J Pharmacol 193:159–163, 1991a

Weiss SRB, Post RM: Development and reversal of conditioned inefficacy and tolerance to the anticonvulsant effects of carbamazepine. Epilepsia 32:140–145, 1991b

Weiss SRB, Post RM: Contingent tolerance to the anticonvulsant effects of carbamazepine, in Carbamazepine: A Bridge Between Epilepsy and Psychiatric Disorders. Edited by Canger E, Perini GI, Sacchetti E, et al. Origgio, Ciba-Geigy Edizioni (in press)

Weiss SRB, Post RM, Patel J, et al: Differential mediation of the anticonvulsant effects of carbamazepine and diazepam. Life Sci 36:2413–2419, 1985

Weiss SRB, Post RM, Gold PW, et al: CRF-induced seizures and behavior: interaction with amygdala kindling. Brain Res 372:345–351, 1986

Weiss SRB, Costello M, Woodward R, et al: Chronic carbamazepine inhibits the development of cocaine-kindled seizures but not its stimulant-induced behavioral sensitization. Abstracts of the Society for Neuroscience, no 262.20, 1987, p 950

Weiss SRB, Post RM, Pert A, et al: Context-dependent cocaine sensitization: differential effect of haloperidol on development versus expression. Pharmacol Biochem Behav 34:655–661, 1989a

Weiss SRB, Post RM, Szele F, et al: Chronic carbamazepine inhibits the development of local anesthetic seizures kindled by cocaine and lidocaine. Brain Res 497:72–79, 1989b

Weiss SRB, Post RM, Costello M, et al: Carbamazepine retards the development of cocaine-kindled seizures but not sensitization to cocaine's effects on hyperactivity and stereotypy. Neuropsychopharmacology 3:273–281, 1990

Weiss SRB, Haas K, Post RM: Contingent tolerance to carbamazepine is associated with lowering of amygdala-kindled seizure thresholds. Exp Neurol 114:300–306, 1991

Winston SM, Hayward MD, Nestler EJ, et al: Chronic electroconvulsive seizures down-regulate expression of the immediate-early genes c-fos and c-jun in rat cerebral cortex. J Neurochem 54:1920–1925, 1990

Wood DM, Lal H: Anxiogenic properties of cocaine withdrawal. Life Sci 41:1431–1436, 1987

Chapter 5

Somatic Manifestations of Normal and Pathological Anxiety

**Rudolf Hoehn-Saric, M.D., and
Daniel R. McLeod, Ph.D.**

N ormal anxiety is a biological warning system that is activated during conditions of potential danger. Because it prepares the body for physical reactions, such as fight or flight, it is accompanied by various bodily changes. In this chapter we shall review the physiological effects of stress- induced anxiety in nonanxious individuals. Further, we shall examine studies dealing with pathological anxiety. The review is limited to physiological states and changes, including those of stress hormones, during psychologically induced arousal. We have omitted pharmacological challenge studies, however, because in those studies it is often difficult to distinguish between the physiological effects of the challenge drug and those of anxiety. Also omitted are hormonal challenge studies, the discussion of which would lengthen the chapter beyond its limits.

MEASUREMENT OF PSYCHOPHYSIOLOGICAL STATES

A full understanding of a person's physiological makeup requires a knowledge of physiological processes when a person is 1) truly relaxed; 2) mildly aroused during the response to standardized stressors, such as difficult mental tasks; and 3) anticipating an unpleasant sensation, such as a painful shock or startle induced by a sudden noise. Further, we should know a person's physiological response to anxiety-provoking situations and, in the case of pathological anxiety, the physiological changes that occur during a disorder-specific syndrome, such as a panic attack. Finally, it is important to know how adaptable a person is. This can be determined by measuring the rate of habituation to innocuous stimuli and the speed of recovery after the termination of a stressful event.

Use of the experimental laboratory to study patients has certain advantages. One can control conditions that by themselves can alter physiological states, such as the environmental temperature, the physical activity of the examined patient, and the exact time of onset for clearly defined stressful situations. Moreover, laboratory examinations permit the recording of multiple physiological systems. The advantage of ambulatory devices, on the other hand, is that they allow us to record the physiological correlates of anxiety in "real life" situations. Several studies have shown that physiological responses in the natural environment exceed those of even very similar situations created in the laboratory (Anderson and Brown 1984; Dimsdale 1984). However, ambulatory recordings are limited by the small number of physiological parameters that can be included, usually heart rate and motility. In addition, these recordings are contaminated by activities unrelated to anxiety and by environmental factors.

Certain bodily activities, such as striated muscle activity, heart rate, blood pressure, and skin conductance, are easily recorded in the laboratory. Other measures, such as respiratory volume and cardiac output, are more cumbersome to record, and their assessment may be taxing to the subject. Even more difficult are examinations of the motility of the gastrointestinal tract, which require special laboratory facilities.

Whereas the recording of muscular activity is usually straightforward, interpretation can be complex. Increased muscular tension is the most frequently reported physiological finding in anxious persons (Hoehn-Saric et al. 1989a). However, not all muscle groups respond equally to anxiety. During baseline measures in the laboratory, forehead muscles usually are found to be more tense (Malmo 1957) but often less responsive to stressors than are other muscle groups (Balshan 1962; Hoehn-Saric et al. 1989a). Muscle tension also varies within the context of an interview. Malmo et al. (1956) demonstrated, in the same patient, increased forearm muscle tension during discussion of hostile conflicts but increased leg muscle tension during discussion of sexual matters.

Most autonomic functions are controlled by the interaction of the sympathetic and parasympathetic nervous systems. An exception is the activity of the eccrine sweat glands, which are controlled entirely by the sympathetic nervous system and whose activity can be assessed through skin conductance measures. However, the sympathetic nervous system is not a uniform system; it consists of a number of functionally separate subdivisions (Hoehn-Saric and McLeod 1988; McCance 1991; Steptoe 1987). The branch that controls sweat gland activity is quite independent from the branch that modifies cardiovascular physiology. Therefore, one cannot draw conclusions about sympathetic activity in other organ systems, such as the heart, on the basis of skin conductance measures. Although we may notice an increase in heart rate, we cannot know a priori whether the change occurred because of an increase in cardiac sympathetic tone or a decrease in cardiac vagal tone, regardless of our knowledge of skin conductance.

To study the effects of anxiety on the subsystems of the autonomic nervous system, one has to employ complex procedures, such as the pharmacological blockade of one of the systems. In spite of these limitations, however, considerable information has been collected on physiological responses to acute stress and chronic anxiety. New techniques, such as improved ambulatory monitors (Thakor et al. 1989) and assessment of vagal tone through power spectral analysis of the oscillations in heart rate associated with respiration (Porges 1986), will permit more accurate measures of not only the functions of organ systems but also the contribution of the individual branches of the autonomic nervous system to these functions.

ACUTE EFFECTS OF STRESS

The effects of anxiety produced by stressful situations have been studied in laboratories and in naturally stressful situations, such as academic examinations, public speaking, pressure at work,

parachute jumping, maneuvering airplanes, anticipating surgery, or dealing with one's dying child (for reviews, see
Frankenhaeuser 1979; Rose 1984; Ursin et al. 1978). The type and
magnitude of bodily responses vary greatly. The most frequently
reported symptoms are increased muscle tension, palpitations,
shortness of breath, lightheadedness, "butterflies in the stom-
ach," increased urinary frequency, and a need to defecate. Ob-
servers may notice dilatation of pupils, paleness of the face,
piloerection, and tremor (Marks 1987). Physiological measures
show increased muscle tension; sympathetic as well as parasympathetic activation; increased secretion of the stress hormones
epinephrine, norepinephrine, cortisol, growth hormone, and prolactin; and decreased secretion of testosterone (Ursin et al. 1978).

Psychophysiological Reactions

The first reaction to a severe fright is parasympathetic: the feeling
of the heart stopping, faintness, and muscle weakness (Gellhorn
1965). Soon, however, the sympathetic system predominates: the
person breaks into a cold sweat, the heart starts to pound, the
limbs shake, and breathing becomes faster and deeper. In less
frightening situations, muscle tension is always increased
(Hoehn-Saric et al. 1989a). The body responds autonomically
with mixed sympathetic-parasympathetic activation. The increased sympathetic tone manifests itself in increased skin conductance corresponding to heightened sweat gland activity.
Heart rate and blood pressure increases are due to sympathetic
activation and possibly to a decrease in vagal tone as well. Urinary and gastrointestinal symptoms, such as a need to urinate,
abdominal discomfort, cramps, and the need to defecate, are
caused by parasympathetic activation (Marks 1987). During
acute stress, persons also tend to breathe more rapidly. The resulting hyperventilation may lead to hypocapnia (an excessive
loss of carbon dioxide in the blood) and thus to respiratory alkalosis. Hypocapnia induces cerebral blood vessel constriction,
which results in feelings of lightheadedness, difficulty articulat-
ing, and, occasionally, fainting. The respiratory alkalosis may
induce muscle cramps and paresthesia around the mouth and the
extremities. Heart rate is frequently increased, and a person may

complain of chest pain. Concomitant swallowing of air may cause abdominal discomfort (for reviews, see Fried 1987; Pincus and Tucker 1985).

Hormonal Reactions

The acute stress response is generally associated with an increased secretion of stress hormones. Norepinephrine is released through the neurosympathetic system, while epinephrine is released through the adrenal medullary gland. Although both hormones are increased under stress, they appear to be differentially activated (Murburg et al. 1990). In the majority of studies, epinephrine has been found to be more responsive to psychological challenges than norepinephrine (Frankenhaeuser 1979; Steptoe 1987). Moreover, postural changes increase norepinephrine levels independently of the anxiety response. Increased excretion of these two hormones, however, is not mood specific and can be seen in all conditions of heightened arousal, such as situations involving novelty and challenges, happy excitement, and anxiety (Frankenhaeuser 1979; Levi 1965). Cortisol increases are more mood specific. Cortisol levels remain low when a challenge is not perceived to be adverse, but they indeed increase during discomfort and anxiety (Frankenhaeuser 1979; Kirschbaum and Hellhammer 1989; Lovallo et al. 1990). Growth hormone and prolactin also increase during stress, but their response is less specific (Nesse et al. 1985).

Personality Traits, Sex, and Stress Response

The autonomic and endocrine responses to a stressor depend on its severity and novelty and on the person's coping ability, personality, sex, and age. Well-adjusted persons tend to have a stronger autonomic and endocrine response to novel situations but adjust faster to harmless situations than do poorly adjusted persons (Frankenhaeuser 1979; Roessler 1973). Women generally have a weaker autonomic response to stressors than do men. During mental stress, for instance, women excrete lower levels of the catecholamines (Frankenhaeuser 1983) and have a weaker systolic blood pressure response than do men (Forsman and Lindblad 1983), in spite of a comparable performance on stressful tasks. The lower sympathetic response to stressors in women may be due to constitutional factors, to cultural and personality factors, or to both. For instance, during college examinations women who were highly competitive with men, such as engineering students, exhibited catecholamine responses similar to those of men and higher than those of women in "traditional" occupations (Frankenhaeuser 1983).

In general, the perception of having some control over a situation lowers autonomic responses to stress (Breier 1989), but this is not always the case (Steptoe 1983). In a study (Frankenhaeuser 1979) in which persons performed arithmetic tasks under noisy conditions, subjects were paired with other subjects in such a way that the first subject, but not the yoked person, could control the noise level. Subjects who rated themselves internally on a locus-of-control scale (Rotter 1966)—that is, persons who regarded themselves as self-reliant—showed a weaker adrenal response when they could control the noise level than when they could not. The opposite was true for persons with an external locus of control—that is, persons who believed that they had little control over their lives and who did not see themselves as being responsible for their destiny. Persons with an external locus of control had a stronger adrenal response when they had to control the noise level and a lower response when they could remain passive.

While personality traits play a role in the intensity of the response to stress, the response depends to a large extent on the perceived importance of the stressor. Williams et al. (1982) demonstrated that autonomic responses to psychological challenges were stronger in competitive Type A persons than in the more easygoing Type B persons. However, Forsman (1980) showed that Type A and Type B persons differed only when the stress was task related; the responses of the two groups were in fact similar when the stress involved problems in interpersonal relationships.

Constitutional Factors and Stress Response

Finally, constitutional factors play an important role in the magnitude of autonomic responses. Several studies have shown that persons who have a positive family history of hypertension exhibit stronger cardiac and blood pressure responses to stress than do persons without such a history (Falkner et al. 1979; Hastrup et al. 1982; Rose and Chesney 1986). Interestingly, mental stressors rather than physical stressors appear to heighten cardiovascular responses in borderline hypertension beyond the increases seen in control subjects (Eliasson 1984). Constitutional factors probably play an important role in the magnitude of response in other body systems, but the relationships between these factors and stress and anxiety are less well understood.

It has been shown that stress can alter motility in practically the entire gastrointestinal tract (Clouse 1988; Ford 1986). Functional abnormalities have been found in the esophagus of persons with esophagospasms and in the colon of persons with irritable bowel syndrome, two conditions that are frequently associated with chronic anxiety. These findings suggest that anxiety may produce strong gastrointestinal changes in a susceptible subpopulation (Clouse 1988). However, because of the difficulties in measuring stress-related gastrointestinal motility, the relationship between perception of a gastrointestinal change and an actual change is poorly understood. (For a discussion of perception of somatic changes versus actual physiological changes, see McLeod and Hoehn-Saric, Chapter 6, this volume.)

The close association of anxiety with somatic manifestations raises questions about the degree to which physiological changes contribute to the overall perception of anxiety. The James-Lange theory (James 1890) actually assumed that the physical response to danger is sufficient to induce the perception of anxiety. This, however, is not always the case. For instance, mitral valve prolapse, which induces episodes of paroxysmal tachycardia, is frequently, but not always, associated with panic disorder (Hickey et al. 1983). This is also true for the irritable bowel syndrome (Clouse 1988). Moreover, neither injections of epinephrine (Cameron et al. 1990a) nor pathological levels of catecholamines in patients with pheochromocytoma (Starkman et al. 1985) lead to heightened anxiety. On the other hand, changes in respiration affect cerebral circulation and may heighten anxiety symptoms (for further discussion, see Post et al., Chapter 4, this volume). Moreover, certain physical changes in anxious persons can become signals that anxiety levels are rising, and these signals can escalate anxiety. To give an example, blushing in a social-phobic subject while meeting someone or the perception of palpitations in a person who delivers a talk can be perceived as loss of control and can trigger severe, sometimes panic-like anxiety.

Physiological Response to Chronic Stress

Chronic stress may or may not lead to adaptation, depending on a person's coping mechanisms. Physiological responses to dangerous activities, such as parachute jumping (Fenz and Epstein 1967; Ursin et al. 1978), show adaptation in well-trained individuals. Similarly, soldiers in Vietnam who were expecting an attack had lower cortisol levels on the day of an attack then during periods immediately before or after. However, the officer in command and the radio operator who carried the burden of responsibility for the decision-making process showed the expected elevation of cortisol (Bourne et al. 1968). On the other hand, situations of chronic distress that do not lead to mastery or the acquisition of coping mechanisms may cause chronic physiological changes.

Elevated blood pressure levels have been found in air traffic controllers (Cobb and Rose 1973) and in persons exposed to noise at work (Jonsson and Hanssen 1977). Also, working women showed higher levels of blood pressure than did homemakers (Kunin and McCormack 1968). A recent survey found higher diastolic blood pressure and left ventricular mass index in persons ages 30 to 40 years with job strain than in subjects without job strain (Schnall et al. 1990). Higher levels of urinary cortisol and urinary catecholamines were associated both with self-reports of physical and mental symptoms and with decrements in test performance in persons living close to Three Mile Island, a nuclear reactor in which an accident involving radiation had occurred several years prior to the study (Schaeffer and Baum 1984).

Thus, it appears that physically healthy persons with appropriate coping resources adapt to chronic stress, while persons with a poor ability to adapt psychologically are more likely to develop physiological changes (Burchfield 1979).

PHYSIOLOGICAL CHANGES IN ANXIETY DISORDERS

Simple Phobias

A simple phobia is a persistent fear of a circumscribed stimulus, object, or situation that almost invariably provokes an immediate anxiety response. Therefore, the object or the situation is avoided or endured with intense anxiety. The person recognizes that his or her fear is excessive or unreasonable (for review, see Marks 1987). In general, persons with simple phobias show no abnormal anxiety in situations that are not related to the specific phobia. Lader et al. (1967) found that subjects with simple phobias were the only anxiety disorder patients they examined whose measurements of electrodermal activity at baseline and during habituation equaled those of nonanxious control subjects. However, when the phobic patients became exposed to a phobic object or situation, they responded physiologically with increased skin conductance, heart rate, and forearm blood flow (Marks 1987; Mathews 1971). Such physiological changes also occurred when a phobic patient only visualized such a situation. Desensitization therapy led to a gradual decrease of the physiological responses. However, psychological, behavioral, and physiological changes did not decrease at an equal pace but instead showed a desynchrony of responses over time (Mathews 1971; Rachman and Hodgson 1974). On the other hand, increased skin conductance response during therapy was found to be associated with a decreased sense of mastery, along with increased symptom experience, symptom occurrence, and negative affect (Glucksman et al. 1985).

Hormonal reactions.   Extensive neuroendocrine studies in phobic patients have been conducted by Curtis and his associates. In one study (Curtis et al. 1976), patients with circumscribed specific phobias were treated with in vivo flooding. Blood samples were drawn every 20 minutes during five separate sessions. The first, second, and fifth sessions were control sessions, while flooding was carried out during the third and fourth sessions. Plasma cortisol secretion followed a general downward curve at each session. The cortisol levels were generally higher during the first and second sessions, suggesting a "novelty" effect rather than a response to anxiety. The authors concluded that adrenal activation may not ordinarily be a part of a phobic reaction or that the chronicity of the phobia allowed the extinction of an earlier adrenal response. In a second study (Curtis et al. 1978), during flooding, the plasma cortisol responses of phobic patients were inconsistent and showed marked individual differences. Only half of the patients responded with increased cortisol secretion in spite of high levels of experienced anxiety. Moreover, when cortisol elevation was associated with flooding, it was usually elevated before, during, and after the confrontation rather than specifically during the confrontation. Flooding in phobic patients led to elevation of plasma growth hormone in some, but not all, patients, and once more the hormonal responses were not related to subjective anxiety (Curtis et al. 1979). In some patients, even intense anxiety failed to stimulate detectable growth hormone secretion. Plasma prolactin levels were not altered by flooding (Nesse et al. 1980). In a recent study, Nesse et al. (1985) reported that in vivo exposure induced significant increases in subjective anxiety, pulse, blood pressure, and plasma levels of norepinephrine, epinephrine, insulin, cortisol, and growth hormone in phobic patients. However, whereas the behavioral manifestations of anxiety were consistent and intense, the magnitude, consistency, timing, and concordance of endocrine and cardiovascular responses showed considerable variations.

Conclusion. Patients with simple phobias do not appear to exhibit higher levels of autonomic arousal than do nonanxious persons, except during exposure to specific phobic objects or situations. During exposure, the phobic patients show increased skin conductance, heart rate, and forearm blood flow. During behavioral treatment, improvement as measured in physiological changes shows a desynchrony from subjective or behavioral changes. Endocrine responses are more complex and highly variable and are not clearly related to anxiety levels during phobic exposure.

Blood-Injury Phobia

Blood-injury phobia is a fear of blood, wounds, or injuries. Exposure to such sights leads to feeling faint and, in some cases, to actual fainting. This disorder is frequently associated with a positive family history and has a high prevalence in the general population (for reviews, see Marks 1988; Thyer et al. 1985). Because blood-injury phobia is a circumscribed disorder that can be studied in the laboratory, its physiology is well documented.

Physiological responses. In contrast to subjects with simple phobias, who show predominantly sympathetic arousal during exposure to phobic situations, individuals with blood-injury phobia exhibit a biphasic physiological response. At first they experience an increase in heart rate and in systolic and diastolic blood pressure; this is followed by a sharp drop in heart rate and blood pressure (Curtis and Thyer 1983; Graham et al. 1961; Öst et al. 1984; Steptoe and Wardle 1988). However, individuals differ greatly in the magnitude and pattern of their physiological response (Steptoe and Wardle 1988). Some patients hyperventilate before and during a procedure such as phlebotomy, thereby inducing hypocapnia (Curtis and Thyer 1983; Ruetz et al. 1967). Patients who faint, or are on the edge of doing so, develop massive bradycardia or a drop in blood pressure, or both. Bradycardia may result in asystole, which is accompanied by apnea (Graham et al. 1961) and which can last up to 25 seconds (Hand and Schröder, cited by Marks 1988). Interestingly, patients with blood-injury phobia do not differ from normal subjects on cardiovascular and respiratory parameters during rest (Steptoe and Wardle 1988) or during physical challenges, such as the cold pressure test, Master's two-step test, or postural change (Ruetz et al. 1967). They respond as other persons do (i.e., with a rise in heart rate) to mental stressors, such as arithmetic or the Stroop color-card test (L. G. Öst, unpublished study, cited by Marks 1988).

The biphasic response of patients with blood-injury phobia to the sight of blood and injury may be explained by an initial sympathetic activation followed by a sudden cessation of sympathetic outflow to the vasoconstrictors and a parasympathetic activation. The initial sympathetic activation manifests itself in increased heart rate and blood pressure, increased vasoconstrictor activity of sympathetic nerves (Wallin and Sundlöf 1982), and possibly increased urinary epinephrine and norepinephrine excretion (Chosy and Graham 1965). However, another study failed to demonstrate an increase in plasma catecholamines prior to phlebotomy (Ruetz et al. 1967). The subsequent drop in heart rate is possibly induced by a sudden increase in the vagal tone, because this response can be blocked with atropine (Menzies 1978). However, in a more recent study, Steptoe and Wardle (1988) used respiratory sinus arrhythmia as a measure of vagal tone in subjects who had fainted during their exposure to a film showing open heart surgery. In spite of a resulting bradycardia, the vagal tone of the subjects did not increase. But, most of the subjects had only a modest bradycardic response to the film. It is possible that marked, but not mild, bradycardia may be associated with increased vagal tone. On the other hand, the drop in blood pressure is associated with a sudden cessation in the outflow of sympathetic vasoconstriction impulses (Wallin and Sundlöf 1982). Therefore, the hypotensive response should not be altered by atropine.

Conclusion.   Blood-injury phobia presents a biphasic cardiovascular response to the sight of blood and injury, consisting of sympathetic activation followed by sudden cessation of sympathetic outflow and, possibly, an increase in vagal tone. Interestingly, the autonomic response, which consists of a sudden drop in heart rate and blood pressure, is limited to blood-related stimuli. The physiological responses of patients with blood-injury phobia to other mental and physical stressors are comparable to those seen in persons who do not suffer from this condition.

Social Phobias

Social phobias may be circumscribed and limited to specific situations, such as speaking or performing in public, or they may have generalized to almost all social situations in which the patient feels under scrutiny and observation. These may include everyday situations such as eating or writing in public, having a social conversation with a member of the opposite sex, or talking to a person of authority. The circumscribed social phobia clinically resembles a simple phobia. The generalized type is frequently associated with high levels of persistent anxiety that resembles generalized anxiety. Patients with social phobias report strong physical responses when they face a feared situation. These responses may include blushing, trembling, choking, and, in severe cases, autonomic symptoms resembling those of panic attacks (for review, see Liebowitz et al. 1985b).

Psychophysiological responses.   No study has measured physiological states of patients with social phobia while these individuals were fully at rest. In a laboratory situation and during a mild challenge, such as listening to repetitive tones, patients with social phobia exhibited elevated electrodermal activity and delayed habituation reactions similar to those seen in agoraphobic patients but unlike those seen in patients with simple phobias or in normal subjects (Lader et al. 1967). This study, however, has not been replicated with patients diagnosed according to more rigorous criteria, such as those of DSM-III-R (American Psychiatric Association 1987). Another study compared volunteers who described themselves as shy and tense in social situations with a group of control subjects during exposure to slides of angry and happy faces and to neutral objects. No difference in skin conductance response or eye blink rate between the groups was found (Merckelbach et al. 1989).

During exposure to specific situations, subjects with social phobia show an increase in heart rate, respiration, and skin conductance (Brady 1984; Johansson and Öst 1982; Lande 1982). Increased heart rate response (Beidel et al. 1985; Heimberg and Barlow 1988; Turner et al. 1986) and a slower-than-normal return to baseline levels (Beidel et al. 1985) have been reported in patients with social phobia during real exposure or while role-playing public speaking.

Hormonal responses.   Stressful public speaking increases plasma epinephrine levels transitorily in normal subjects (Dimsdale and Moss 1980). However, a study that compared subjects with social phobia with normal subjects while these individuals were giving a speech in the laboratory found no difference in heart rate, plasma epinephrine, norepinephrine, or cortisol between the groups (A. Levin, unpublished data, cited by Schneier and Liebowitz 1990).

Heterogeneity of responses. Not all subjects with social phobias respond uniformly to social stressors. Öst et al. (1981) exposed outpatients with social phobias to a social interaction test and monitored heart rate continuously. The authors were able to divide their patients into two groups according to the heart rate response. These two groups subsequently were exposed to two different treatment modalities. One treatment modality focused on social skills training and the other on relaxation. Patients with high heart rates responded more readily to relaxation techniques than to social skills training, whereas the opposite was true for the group with lower heart rates. Thus, it appears that subjects with social phobias differ in psychological and physiological responses.

Conclusion. Social phobias may occur in isolation or may be generalized to multiple social situations. The differences in physiological response patterns between the two groups have not been fully explored. The physiological states of subjects with social phobias who are relaxed have not been studied. One study reported that, in the laboratory, subjects with social phobias exhibited greater fluctuations in electrodermal activity and slower habituation than did subjects with simple phobias or normal subjects. This finding suggests increased sympathetic tone. When exposed to feared situations, subjects with social phobias exhibit higher than normal skin conductance, heart rate, and respiration frequency. However, stress hormones do not appear to be excessively elevated during phobic situations, and the physiological responses to stressful situations are comparatively small. Therefore, Schneier and Liebowitz (1990) suggested that "social phobics appear to suffer from an exaggerated awareness rather than an increased amount of peripheral autonomic arousal" (p. 171).

Posttraumatic Stress Disorder

Posttraumatic stress disorder (PTSD) is an anxiety disorder resulting from an event that is outside of the usual human experience and one that would be markedly distressing to almost anyone. PTSD partially resembles a grief reaction: the patient is plagued by recurrent and intrusive recollections of the stressful event as well as recurring distressing dreams, and he or she may experience dissociation. PTSD also resembles a phobia—namely, the experience of intense distress, sometimes resembling that seen during panic attacks, when exposed to events that symbolize or resemble an aspect of the traumatic event. This response then leads to resistance to face such events and to avoidance of such situations. In addition, PTSD patients often suffer from chronic anxiety, dysphoria, or depression (for reviews, see Giller 1990; Wolf and Mosnaim 1990).

Most studies on PTSD were conducted on war veterans. This is unfortunate, because PTSD that occurs frequently in civilian life may differ from the clinical manifestations seen in veterans (Davidson et al. 1990). When assessing PTSD, one has to keep in mind that only some persons who were exposed to traumatic situations subsequently develop a chronic form of PTSD. The cause of heightened vulnerability in this subpopulation remains unknown. Introversion, neuroticism, and a past history and family history of psychiatric disorders have been found to be associated with the development of chronic PTSD (McFarlane 1988).

Only a few psychophysiological studies on PTSD have been designed with the same methodological rigor as the more numerous studies on panic disorder. However, these few studies present interesting findings, which are summarized below.

Psychophysiological and hormonal states at "baseline." No study has measured physiological states of PTSD patients while these individuals were truly relaxed. During baseline measures in the laboratory, Dobbs and Wilson (1960) found no difference in heart rate but a higher respiratory rate in "decompensated" as compared with "compensated" combat veterans. Malloy et al. (1983) detected no difference between combat veterans with and without PTSD on baseline recordings of heart rate or skin resistance. Blanchard et al. (1982) compared combat veterans who had PTSD with an age-matched noncombat control group and found the PTSD patients to have higher heart rates but not higher systolic blood pressures. In a second study, which compared combat veterans with and without PTSD, Blanchard et al. (1986) found higher heart rates in PTSD patients at baseline. Pitman et al. (1987) compared veterans who reacted differently to similar combat experiences. One group of veterans had developed PTSD, whereas the other had not. The authors found differences in heart rate, but not differences in skin conductance or electromyographic recordings, between the two groups. McFall et al. (1990) compared veterans who had PTSD with a somewhat mixed controlled group and found no difference between the groups on heart rate, blood pressure, or plasma epinephrine or norepinephrine.

Physiological responses to stimuli unrelated to trauma.   When exposed to stimuli that were not related to the original trauma— for instance, neutral videotapes (Malloy et al. 1983), films of car accidents (McFall et al. 1990), mental arithmetic alone (Blanchard et al. 1982, 1986), arithmetic plus startle sounds (Pallmeyer et al. 1986), or listening to a "neutral script" (Pitman et al. 1987)— PTSD patients did not react differently physiologically than control subjects. Interestingly, PTSD patients actually had less of an increase on the forehead electromyogram (EMG) during mental arithmetic than did control subjects (Blanchard et al. 1982) and exhibited smaller physiological responses (type of response not specified) to the listening of a mental script (Pitman et al. 1987).

Physiological responses to trauma-related stimuli.   Responses to stimuli that were related to the traumatic experience, such as combat sounds (Blanchard et al. 1982, 1986; Dobbs and Wilson 1960; Pallmeyer et al. 1986), videotapes of combat (Malloy et al. 1983), or listening to a combat-related script (Pitman et al. 1987), uniformly produced higher subjective and physiological responses in PTSD patients than in control subjects. In the study by Dobbs and Wilson (1960), the patients became so disturbed during the exposure that it became impossible to record physiological measures. Malloy et al. (1983), Blanchard et al. (1982, 1986), Pallmeyer et al. (1986), and McFall et al. (1990) reported higher heart rates in PTSD patients during exposure. In addition, higher skin resistance response (Malloy et al. 1983), forehead EMG, systolic blood pressure (Blanchard et al. 1986), and diastolic blood pressure, but not plasma epinephrine or norepinephrine levels (McFall et al. 1990), were found in PTSD patients. McFall et al. (1990) also noticed in PTSD patients a slower recovery of heart rate, blood pressure, and epinephrine levels after exposure.

Hormonal responses to stressors. The results of urinary hormonal studies are more difficult to evaluate because urine was collected over 24 hours that included periods of rest and sleep as well as heightened arousal and physical activity. Moreover, several studies used control groups consisting of patients with major mental illnesses. Higher epinephrine and norepinephrine levels were reported in PTSD patients in one study (Kosten et al. 1987), suggesting that these patients have higher sympathetic tone; however, cortisol output was found to be lower in patients with PTSD than in patients with major depression or schizophrenia (Mason et al. 1986). The latter finding was confirmed in a study that compared PTSD patients with nonpsychiatric subjects (Yehuda et al. 1990). The authors believed that the results presented a physiological adaptation of the hypothalamo-pituitary-adrenocortical axis to chronic stress. The mechanism of this adaptation is not well understood but may involve psychological (Mason et al. 1986) as well as physiological mechanisms (Odio and Brodish 1990). Not all studies have found differences between PTSD patients and patients with a major mental illness on urinary catecholamine or cortisol levels. However, as a group, PTSD patients had a higher norepinephrine/cortisol ratio than did other patient groups (Mason et al. 1988).

Only a few studies have examined physiological changes in patients who acquired PTSD in noncombat situations. Kozak et al. (cited by Orr 1990) asked rape victims to imagine a standardized sexual assault situation and found no significant increases in heart rate or skin conductance response in rape victims when compared with a control group.

Conclusion.   Most studies of PTSD have been conducted in clinically ill combat veterans. No information is available on whether PTSD patients are hyperaroused under resting conditions. During baseline measures, several but not all studies reported increased heart rate. With the exception of respiratory rates, other physiological parameters were not elevated. Noncombat-related stimuli induced physiological changes in PTSD patients that were similar or weaker to those found in control subjects. These findings suggest that PTSD patients do not overreact indiscriminately to stimuli and, at times, are less involved in interactions that are unrelated to their psychopathology than are control subjects. All studies are in agreement, however, that clinically ill combat veterans overreact to trauma-related stimuli and that PTSD patients recover more slowly from such provocations. Hormonal studies are difficult to interpret, but they do not suggest excessive excretion of stress hormones.

Controlled studies of PTSD patients who are not war veterans would be helpful in broadening our knowledge of this disorder. Presently, most data are derived from a group of patients who, for unknown reasons, respond excessively in magnitude and duration to traumatic situations that others are quite capable of overcoming. Finding the reasons as to why some individuals, but not others, exhibit such vulnerability will greatly advance our knowledge of this interesting disorder.

Generalized Anxiety Disorder

Generalized anxiety disorder (GAD) is the most common anxiety disorder (Weissman 1985). Therefore, it is surprising how little study has been devoted to it. GAD is characterized by unrealistic or excessive anxiety and worry about life circumstances and is frequently accompanied by physical symptoms, such as muscle tension, autonomic hyperactivity, and vigilance (for review, see Hoehn-Saric and McLeod 1990).

Psychophysiological states and response patterns.   Because GAD tends to be chronic, one would expect to find physiological differences between patients with GAD and control subjects. We do not have data on GAD patients when they are truly at rest.

However, when we (Hoehn-Saric et al. 1989a) examined GAD patients (who had never had panic attacks) in the laboratory, we found that only higher forehead and gastrocnemius muscle tension distinguished them physiologically from nonanxious control subjects. Skin conductance, heart rate, and respiration levels were comparable to those levels in nonanxious persons. During performance of stressful mental tasks, such as a divided attention task and a computerized game in which the participant wins or loses money, GAD patients and control subjects showed similar physiological changes, except that the skin conductance and heart rate ranges were smaller in patients than in control subjects. These smaller ranges indicate a narrower range of autonomic responsivity during laboratory stress. We have obtained similar results in a population of patients who were retrospectively diagnosed as having had GAD (Hoehn-Saric and Masek 1981).

Clinically, GAD patients do not form a homogeneous group. Different patient groups complain of different symptom clusters. These symptoms are generally muscular, cardiovascular, or gastrointestinal (Weiner 1985). Therefore, it is possible that groups of GAD patients also differ in their physiological responses. We (Hoehn-Saric et al. 1989b) compared a group of GAD patients who expressed high levels of cardiac complaints with a group who expressed low levels of such complaints. The two groups were comparable on measures of psychic anxiety, but they differed physiologically. Patients with high levels of cardiac complaints had higher levels of skin conductance at rest and showed greater cardiac variability during the stress tasks. However, studies examining physiological differences between GAD patients with high and low levels of gastrointestinal complaints have not been conducted.

Hormonal states.   Hormonal studies have generally failed to show differences between GAD patients and control subjects. Rosenbaum et al. (1983) examined urinary cortisol levels in GAD outpatients, and we (Hoehn-Saric et al. 1991a) studied plasma cortisol levels during baseline and laboratory stress. Neither study found cortisol levels to differ between patients and control subjects.

Several studies have examined plasma catecholamines.

Mathew et al. (1981) reported increased plasma epinephrine and norepinephrine levels in one study but were unable to reproduce these findings in another study (Mathew et al. 1982). The authors attributed the positive results of the first study to a premature withdrawal of the blood sample after venipuncture. Munjack et al. (1990) found no differences in plasma levels of epinephrine, norepinephrine, or 3-methoxy-4-hydroxyphenylglycol (MHPG) between GAD patients and control subjects. Peronnet et al. (1986) also found no differences in epinephrine or norepinephrine levels when they compared students with high and low levels of trait anxiety. Only a study by Sevy et al. (1989) reported significant differences between patients and control subjects on plasma norepinephrine and MHPG levels.

Conclusion. It appears that in spite of subjective somatic complaints, patients with GAD are physiologically similar to nonanxious persons at rest. In laboratory findings only heightened muscle tension differentiates GAD patients from normal subjects. Under laboratory stress, the degree of response in GAD patients is comparable to that in normal subjects, except that the range of autonomic responsiveness in GAD patients is narrower. However, GAD patients do not form a homogeneous group, and subgroups may differ in their responses to stress. Stress hormone levels appear to be within the normal range, although some subgroups may have a higher catecholamine output.

Physiological studies of GAD patients during their responses to everyday stressors and during heightened anxiety in a natural environment have not been conducted. Therefore, it is unknown whether GAD patients respond differently physiologically than nonanxious persons to "real life" situations.

Panic Disorder

Panic disorder is characterized by paroxysmal attacks of anxiety accompanied by strong somatic, particularly cardiovascular and respiratory, reactions (for review, see Ballenger 1990a, 1990b).

Physiological states at baseline. There is no evidence that panic disorder patients suffer from cardiac hyperactivity when they are truly at rest. Four studies using cardiac monitors (Freedman et al. 1985; Shear 1986; Taylor et al. 1983, 1986) found no differences between panic disorder patients and control subjects when the patients were not tense. One study found increases in the number of premature ventricular contractions experienced by panic disorder subjects during periods of increased anxiety (Shear et al. 1987). However, a second study showed no increase in heart rate during anticipatory anxiety (Taylor et al. 1986).

The physiological "baseline" measures obtained in the laboratory on panic disorder patients and control subjects are summarized in Table 5–1. Because an examination in a laboratory usually induces a mild degree of distress, baseline measures do not reflect a truly relaxed state. In most studies, patients had been drug free for an adequate period at the time of testing. Baseline measures were usually taken before the performance of a task or a challenge test. About one-third of the studies found that panic disorder patients exhibited heightened heart rates and increased systolic blood pressure, and slightly more than one-quarter of the studies found increased diastolic blood pressure. Skin conductance was elevated in two studies (Roth et al. 1986, 1990) and showed a trend toward significance in another study (Hoehn-Saric et al. 1991b). One study (Hoehn-Saric et al. 1991b) reported elevated forehead muscle tension. Several, but not all, studies found physiological evidence of hyperventilation during baseline (Gorman et al. 1986, 1988; Woods et al. 1988). Interestingly, in none of the studies were stress hormones found to be elevated, except in a study by Villacres et al. (1987), and this study has been criticized on methodological grounds (Papp et al. 1988).

Physiological responses to nonspecific stressors. We (Hoehn-Saric et al. 1991b) found that exposure of panic disorder patients to psychological stressors led to a greater increase in systolic blood pressure but to a narrower range in skin conductance than was found in nonanxious control subjects. Yaragani et al. (1990a, 1991) also reported decreased R-R variance in the electrocardiogram of panic disorder patients compared with control subjects. Two studies that measured habituation to auditory stimuli reported a slower habituation of skin conductance in the panic disorder group than in control subjects (Lader et al. 1967; Roth et

Table 5–1. Physiological baseline measures in panic disorder patients: comparison with normal control subjects

Study	Subjects[a]	Drug-free period	Baseline before challenge[b]	Measures[c]
Cardiovascular measures				
Cameron et al. (1990a)	24 PD 32 C	10 days +	None	HR = SBP = DBP =
Charney and Heninger (1986)	26 PD 21 C	21 days +	Clonidine	HR ↑ SBP ↑ DBP =
Charney et al. (1984)	39 PD 20 C	21 days +	Yohimbine	HR = SBP = DBP =
Charney et al. (1985)	21 PD 17 C	21 days +	Caffeine	HR = SBP = DBP =
Charney et al. (1987)	23 PD 19 C	21 days +	m-CPP	HR = SBP = DBP =
Cowley et al. (1987)	44 PD 10 C	14 days +	Sodium lactate	HR = SBP ↑ DBP ↑
Freedman et al. (1985)	12 PD 11 C	14 days +	Ambulatory monitor	HR = when not tense
Gaffney et al (1988)	10 PD 10 C	14 days +	Sodium lactate	HR = SBP = DBP =
Gorman et al. (1988)	31 PD 13 C	28 days +	Hyperventilation	HR ↑ SBP ↑ DBP ↑
Hoehn-Saric et al. (1991b)	18 PD 18 C	21 days +	Psychological stressor	HR ↑ SBP ↑ DBP =
Holden and Barlow (1986)	10 PD 10 C	Some patients on anxiolytics	Exposure	HR ↑
Liebowitz et al. (1985a)	43 PD 20 C	3 days +	Sodium lactate	HR ↑ SBP = DBP ↑
Roth et al. (1986)	37 PD 19 C	Some patients on medications	Tones	HR ↑

Table 5–1. Physiological baseline measures in panic disorder patients: comparison with normal control subjects *(continued)*

Study	Subjects[a]	Drug-free period	Baseline before challenge[b]	Measures[c]
Taylor et al. (1987)	40 PD 40 C	14 days +	Treadmill	HR =
Weissman et al. (1987)	37 PD 33 C	3 days +	Postural, valsalva	HR = SBP = DBP =
Woods et al. (1987)	18 PD 13 C	28 days +	Exposure	HR = SBP ↑ DBP =
Woods et al. (1988)	14 PD 11 C	35 days +	CO_2	HR = SBP = DBP =
Yaragani et al. (1989)	61 PD 25 C	14 days +	Sodium lactate	HR = SBP = DBP =
Yaragani et al. (1990b)	30 PD 30 C	14 days +	Postural, isometric	HR = SBP = DBP ↑

Respiratory measures

Study	Subjects[a]	Drug-free period	Baseline before challenge[b]	Measures[c]
Gaffney et al. (1988)	10 PD 10 C	14 days +	Sodium lactate	R =
Gorman et al. (1985)	21 PD 10 C	Not stated	Sodium lactate	pCO_2 = Bicarbonates = Venous pH more variable
Gorman et al. (1986)	76 PD 22 C	14 days +	Sodium lactate	pCO_2 ↓ Bicarbonates ↓ Venous pH ↑
Gorman et al. (1988)	31 PD 13 C	28 days +	Hyperventilation	pCO_2 = Tidal volumes ↑
Hoehn-Saric et al. (1991b)	18 PD 18 C	21 days +	Psychological stressor	R =
Holt and Andrews (1989)	50 PD 16 C	Not stated	Hyperventilation	pCO_2 =
Liebowitz et al. (1985a)	43 PD 20 C	3 days +	Sodium lactate	pCO_2 = Bicarbonate =

Table 5–1.   Physiological baseline measures in panic disorder patients: comparison with normal control subjects (*continued*)

Study	Subjects[a]	Drug-free period	Baseline before challenge[b]	Measures[c]
Woods et al. (1988)	14 PD 11 C	35 days +	CO_2	R ↑
Electrodermal activity				
Hoehn-Saric et al. (1991b)	18 PD 18 C	21 days +	Psychological stressor	SC mean = Range = Variability =
Roth et al. (1986)	37 PD 10 C	Some patients on medication	Tones	SC mean ↑ SC fluct ↑
Roth et al. (1990)	38 PD 22 C	14 days +	Tones Psychological stressor Hyperventilation	SC mean ↑ SC fluct ↑
Muscular activity				
Hoehn-Saric et al. (1991b)	18 PD 18 C	21 days +	Psychological stimuli	FEMG = ↑ GEMG =
Stress hormones				
Cameron et al. (1990a)	24 PD 32 C	10 days +	None	E = NE =
Charney and Heninger (1986)	26 PD 21 C	21 days +	Clonidine	MHPG = Cortisol = GH =
Charney et al. (1984)	39 PD 20 C	21 days +	Yohimbine	MHPG =
Charney et al. (1985)	21 PD 17 C	21 days +	Caffeine	MHPG = Cortisol =
Charney et al. (1987)	23 PD 19 C	21 days +	m-CPP	Cortisol = GH = PL =
Gaffney et al. (1988)	10 PD 10 C	14 days +	Sodium lactate	E = NE =
Kathol et al. (1988)	65 PD 11 C	7 days +	None	24-hour urine Cortisol =
Levin et al. (1987)	17 PD 5 C	14 days +	Sodium lactate	Cortisol = ACTH =

Table 5–1. Physiological baseline measures in panic disorder patients: comparison with normal control subjects (*continued*)

Study	Subjects[a]	Drug-free period	Baseline before challenge[b]	Measures[c]
Liebowitz et al. (1985a)	43 PD 20 C	3 days +	Sodium lactate	E = NE = Cortisol = PL =
Papp et al. (1988)	24 PD 8 C	3 days +	Sodium lactate CO_2	Arterial E =
Pohl et al. (1987)	10 PD 9 C	14 days +	Sodium lactate Isoproterenol	MHPG =
Rapaport et al. (1989)	8 PD 8 C	14 days +	CRH	Cortisol = ACTH =
Schneider et al. (1987)	8 PD 11 C	Some patients on benzodiazepines	Postural	E = NE =
Uhde et al. (1988)	12 PD 12 C	14 days +	None	Urinary MHPG = Urinary cortisol =
Villacres et al. (1987)	10 PD 10 C	14 days +	None	Arterialized venous blood E = ↑ NE = Cortisol =
Woods et al. (1987)	18 PD 13 C	28 days +	Exposure	MHPG = Cortisol = GH = PL =
Woods et al. (1988)	14 PD 11 C	35 days +	CO_2	MHPG = Cortisol = GH = PL =

Note. ↑/↓ means measure differs significantly from the control group. "=" indicates measure does not differ from control group. All stress hormones were assessed from venous samples unless noted otherwise.
[a]PD = panic disorder patients; C = normal control subjects.
[b]m-CPP = *m*-chlorophenylpiperazine.
[c]HR = heart rate; SBP = systolic blood pressure; DBP = diastolic blood pressure; R = respiration rate; SC = skin conductance; FEMG = forehead electromyogram; GEMG = gastrocnemius electromyogram; E = epinephrine; NE = norepinephrine; MHPG = 3-methoxy-4-hydroxyphenylglycol; GH = growth hormone; PL = prolactin.

al. 1990). Physiological challenges, such as postural changes, Valsalva maneuver, or treadmill exercise, generally induced stronger cardiovascular responses in panic disorder patients than in control subjects (Gaffney et al. 1988; Schneider et al. 1987; Taylor et al. 1987; Weissman et al. 1987; Yaragani et al. 1989). These changes were interpreted as signs of increased autonomic cardiovascular lability in panic disorder, but they also could have been attributed to lower physical fitness.

Physiological responses to panic attacks.   The recording of a full range of physiological parameters during a spontaneous panic attack is technically difficult. The occurrence of panic attacks is sporadic and unpredictable, and ambulatory devices are limited in their recording capacity. Therefore, only limited information is available on the physiology of naturally occurring panic attacks. Lader and Mathews (1970) recorded physiological changes in three patients who developed spontaneous panic attacks during a recording session. The attacks were associated with a sudden increase (of up to 50 beats per minute) in heart rate, along with increases in skin conductance, finger pulse volume, and forearm blood flow. Interestingly, the forearm EMG did not change. Patients' physiological states normalized gradually within several minutes. Sudden heart rate elevation in two patients who developed spontaneous panic attacks in the laboratory was also reported by Cohen et al. (1985). Balon et al. (1988) reported significant heart rate and systolic and diastolic blood pressure increases in patients who panicked during a placebo (dextrose) infusion.

Studies using ambulatory monitors (Freedman et al. 1985; Shear et al. 1987; Taylor et al. 1983, 1986) also reported heart rate changes associated with panic attacks. However, not all panic attacks were accompanied by an increase in heart rate. During panic attacks, an increased number of premature ventricular contractions occur, but similar cardiac rhythm disturbances occur also during periods of heightened nonpanic anxiety (Shear et al. 1987). Moreover, the frequency of arrhythmias during anxiety and during panic attacks does not exceed generally acceptable limits.

The most comprehensive study of nonpharmacologically induced panic attacks was conducted by Woods et al. (1987). The authors provoked situational panic attacks in 15 out of 18 panic disorder patients by exposing them to situations in which these patients frequently panicked. During the attacks, patients' heart rates increased but their blood pressures and plasma levels of MHPG, cortisol, growth hormone, and prolactin remained within the prepanic range. On the other hand, Ko et al. (1983) found that plasma MHPG levels were elevated 30 minutes after panic attacks induced in patients by exposure to a phobic situation.

Physiological responses to behavioral interactions. Studies that monitored cardiac responses to behavioral interventions in agoraphobic patients (Holden and Barlow 1986; Mavissakalian and Michelson 1982) reported that increased heart rate accompanied heightened anxiety during exposure (e.g., a walk through an open area). As treatment progressed, clinical manifestation and heart rate decreased. However, subjective and behavioral manifestations responded earlier than heart rate, demonstrating the desynchrony that has been observed during behavior therapy of simple phobias. In one study (Craske et al. 1987), increased heart rate was associated with a good outcome because patients who were willing to approach feared situations responded with a greater increase in heart rate to the exposure than did hesitant, nonassertive patients.

Conclusion. The only evidence that panic disorder patients are autonomically hyperaroused when they are not anxious comes from resting conditions in the laboratory, and these data have not been supported by studies using ambulatory monitors. Mild stressors have led to increased heart rate and blood pressure in some, but not all, studies. These discrepancies between studies may be attributed to differences in the patients' expectations when anticipating pharmacological challenges or testing. Some challenges, such as mental and physical tasks, are mildly stressful, and pharmacological challenges that are given to induce a panic attack can be quite distressing. However, as seen in Table 5–1, the anticipation of a stressful challenge alone does not explain the differences. The differences may be caused by methodological problems, including the choice of control groups. Most likely, however, physiological manifestations are related to the severity of the panic disorder. Clinically, patients with infrequent panic attacks appear less distressed than patients with frequent panic attacks (Uhde et al. 1985). Patients in the latter group often complain of high levels of tension, even when they are free of panic attacks, and this tension is independent of the anticipatory anxiety. Charney et al. (1984) found that only patients with frequent panic attacks had an enhanced physiological response to yohimbine challenge; patients with less frequent panic attacks did not differ from the control subjects in their response. Beck and Scott (1988) also found that patients with frequent panic attacks had significantly higher trapezius EMG levels than did patients with infrequent panic attacks. Our study (Hoehn-Saric et al. 1991b), which examined only patients with frequent panic attacks, also found differences in heart rate and systolic blood pressure between patients and nonanxious control subjects. Heightened cardiorespiratory responses to psychological and pharmacological stimuli in patients who have frequent panic attacks (Ballenger 1989) may be related to the severity of the disorder.

Interestingly, in spite of a cardiovascular hyperactivity of our patients during baseline and stress tasks, panic disorder patients, like GAD and OCD patients, exhibited a restricted skin conductance response (Hoehn-Saric et al. 1991b). Moreover, panic disorder patients habituate more slowly than normal control subjects to innocuous stimuli (e.g., tones) (Lader 1967; Roth et al. 1986, 1990). Thus, panic disorder patients, like patients with other chronic anxiety disorders, exhibit diminished autonomic flexibility.

The role of the autonomic nervous system in the initiation of panic attacks remains unclear. Most investigators believe that sudden sympathetic changes initiate panic attacks. An alternative explanation—namely, a sudden decrease in vagal tone—has been suggested by Shear (1986) and has been shown to occur during hyperventilation in normal subjects (George et al. 1989). However, this decrease in vagal tone has not been studied in patients with panic attacks.

Some, but not all, panic disorder patients hyperventilate, even during baseline recording. Thus, a subgroup of patients may be chronic hyperventilators. In many patients, hyperventilation probably does not induce panic attacks (Gorman et al. 1988; Hibbert and Pilsbury 1989), but it may lower the threshold for an attack. Some investigators, however, believe that hyperventilation may be the cause of all (Ley 1985; Lum 1975), or at least some (Bass et al. 1987), panic attacks.

Finally, one has to keep in mind that a large number of panic disorder patients suffer from mitral valve prolapse, a condition that by itself is associated with heightened sympathetic activity and manifests itself in episodes of palpitations and arrhythmias (Davies et al. 1987). Also, inner ear problems causing dizziness are found in a subgroup of panic disorder patients (Jacob 1988) and may further complicate the physiology of panic disorder.

The fact that only one study found an elevation in stress hormones at baseline suggests either an absence of chronic hyperarousal or an adaptation to a long-standing disorder. The hormonal response to situational panic attacks appears to be as unpredictable as that seen in simple phobias.

In general, the physiological responses to panic attacks are surprisingly low in magnitude when one considers how intense the subjective experiences are. Frequently, a physiological response may even be absent. On the other hand, in some patients, panic attacks are accompanied by dramatic cardiovascular changes (Lader and Mathews 1970). Such patients may be constitutionally predisposed toward excessive cardiovascular responses. The coexistence of mitral valve prolapse may further complicate a patient's condition. Moreover, in patients who suffer from a cardiovascular disease, even limited physiological changes during stress, including a panic attack, may suffice to induce ischemia or serious arrhythmias (Rozanski et al. 1988). Therefore, a subgroup of panic disorder patients are at high risk for premature death due to cardiovascular diseases (Coryell et al. 1982; Weissman et al. 1990).

Obsessive-Compulsive Disorder

Obsessive-compulsive disorder (OCD) is classified by DSM-III-R as an anxiety disorder, but investigators are unable to agree on its proper categorization (Insel et al. 1985). Most researchers agree, however, that anxiety plays an important contributory role in

OCD. Anxiety in OCD patients occurs during obsessive thoughts, particularly when the thoughts anticipate potential harm. Anxiety is also heightened when patients try to control their compulsive urges. In addition, GAD-like anxiety is often present independently of OCD symptoms. We found that on anxiety scales, OCD patients, as a group, produce scores similar to those of GAD patients. Some patients report panic-like attacks, but these attacks are more likely to be associated with obsessions or compulsions than to occur spontaneously (for review, see Jenike et al. 1990).

Physiological states of baseline and responses to stressors. Physiological states of OCD patients during a true state of rest have not been studied. During baseline measures in the laboratory, OCD patients do not differ from control subjects on heart rate or skin conductance (Boulougouris 1977; Hoehn-Saric et al. 1988), but, like patients with other anxiety disorders, OCD patients do exhibit higher levels of muscle tension (Hoehn-Saric et al. 1988). During psychological stress tasks, OCD patients show autonomic responses similar to those of normal control subjects, except that their skin conductance and heart interbeat interval range are diminished and their systolic blood pressure is increased (Hoehn-Saric et al. 1988). On the other hand, distressing stimuli, such as a painful electric shock, produce greater skin conductance and heart rate responses in OCD patients than in control subjects (Beech and Liddell 1974).

Physiological responses to illness-specific situations. When OCD patients were exposed to illness-specific situations, they exhibited increased heart rate and skin conductance. These responses diminished in intensity as behavioral treatment progressed (Boulougouris et al. 1977). As was the case for phobic patients who underwent desensitization, behavioral treatment of OCD patients led to a desynchrony between subjective, behavioral, and autonomic responses (Hodgson and Rachman 1972; Lelliott et al. 1987). A problem in the assessment of physiological responses to OCD-specific stimuli in the laboratory is the fact that not all OCD symptoms are readily induced outside of a patient's home. Whereas phobic-like fears of contamination can be induced everywhere, compulsive checking behavior tends to occur mainly in circumscribed situations; therefore, "checkers" do not produce OCD-specific responses in the laboratory (Rachman and Hodgson 1980).

Urinary cortisol levels in patients with OCD appear to be within the normal range; however, they tend to increase more during therapeutic exposure than during control sessions (Kasvikis et al. 1988).

Conclusion. In summary, typical OCD patients do not appear to be hyperaroused when at rest. During mild tension, such as during baseline recording in the laboratory, they show physiological responses similar to those seen in GAD patients, that is, increased muscle tension but no autonomic hyperactivity. When exposed to nonspecific mental stressors, they exhibit responses similar to those seen in GAD patients, namely, physiological changes similar in magnitude to but smaller in range than those of control subjects. However, the response of OCD patients to adverse stimuli, such as an electric shock, appears to be increased. OCD patients also show an increased response to disorder-specific stimuli (e.g., obsessive thoughts and compulsions). These responses gradually decrease with successful behavior therapy. Cortisol levels do not appear to be elevated at rest but tend to increase at times of confrontation with symptom-specific situations.

DIMINISHED AUTONOMIC FLEXIBILITY

Diminished autonomic flexibility has been shown to occur in various conditions of social maladaptation, including chronic anxiety. Lader and Wing (1964) found that nonanxious subjects had larger galvanic skin responses to novel stimuli but habituated faster than patients with anxiety states. Kelly (1980) reported greater forearm blood flow increases during mental stress in normal subjects than in anxiety patients. These findings are consistent with reports by Forsman (1980) and Frankenhaeuser (1979), who found that persons with stable personalities had stronger catecholamine responses to stressors than did poorly adjusted persons or persons with high levels of neuroticism.

After termination of stress, catecholamines returned to previous levels more rapidly in well-adjusted than in ill-adjusted persons. Similar to the skin conductance response, the catecholamine response to stress was initially weaker but more prolonged in persons with poor adjustment.

We found diminished flexibility in cardiac and skin conductance responses during mental stress in GAD (Hoehn-Saric et al. 1989a) and OCD (Hoehn-Saric et al. 1988) patients and diminished range of responses in skin conductance in panic disorder patients (Hoehn-Saric et al. 1991b). Yaragani et al. (1990a, 1991) reported decreased R-R variability in the electrocardiogram of panic disorder patients. Slower habituation to tones has also been observed in panic disorder patients (Lader 1967; Roth et al. 1986, 1990).

Central nervous system measures support decreased reactivity to nonspecific stressors in persons with heightened anxiety. Tecce (1972) showed that anxiety reduces contingent negative variation amplitude, while Grillon and Buchsbaum (1987) found that GAD patients had less of a decrease in alpha activity during light stimulation than did normal control subjects. Thus, well-adjusted persons exhibit a stronger but more flexible response to stress and gain autonomic equilibrium faster than do those individuals with poor adjustment or with high levels of chronic anxiety. However, diminished flexibility may also lead to inappropriate, excessive responses when the stressors are perceived as anxiety producing or are pathology specific. Such excessive and prolonged responses can be observed in phobic patients and in PTSD patients.

There are several, not mutually exclusive, explanations for this phenomenon. Obviously, diminished autonomic flexibility is not disorder specific. It does not represent merely a "ceiling effect," that is, a continuously high level of physiological arousal that permits only a modest further increase under stress. This explanation may be applicable to some conditions (Kelly 1980), but, in general, baseline values of anxiety patients differ little from those of nonanxious control subjects.

Another, not yet fully explored possibility is that diminished autonomic flexibility represents a constitutional weakness that renders a person vulnerable to the development of maladaptive conditions, including anxiety disorders. Studies of shy children by Kagan et al. (1988) suggest that this may be the case in some patients. This phenomenon may also represent a partial but inadequate attempt by the body to adapt to the physiological changes induced by anxiety (Burchfield 1979).

Finally, a psychological explanation is plausible. The heightened preoccupation of patients with their internal events may diminish their attention to stimuli that are unrelated to their pathology (see McLeod and Hoehn-Saric, Chapter 6, this volume). For instance, some PTSD patients showed less of a physiological response than control subjects when they listened to a neutral script (Pitman et al. 1987) or mental arithmetic (Blanchard et al. 1982), but they overresponded to trauma-related stimuli. Shapiro and Crider (1969), who reviewed the older literature, concluded that "organized attempts to cope with environmental threats are accompanied by autonomic reactivity, whereas disorganization and defensiveness are correlated with reduced autonomic involvement" (pp. 35–36). Thus, chronic anxiety patients respond to tension-inducing tasks with a physiological response that is smaller in magnitude but longer in duration. Their response to noxious and pathology-specific stimuli, however, is excessive as well as prolonged. Both types of responses are congruent with the concept of diminished autonomic flexibility.

CONCLUSIONS

Acute anxiety produces distinct physiological changes in nonanxious persons as well as in patients with anxiety disorders. In nonanxious persons, changes depend on the type and severity of the stressor, on the perception of the stressor, and on a person's age, sex, personality, and constitution. Physiological responses consist of increased muscle tension, autonomic changes that are induced by increased or decreased sympathetic and parasympathetic activity, increased secretion of stress hormones, and decreased secretion of testosterone. The magnitude and pattern of physiological responses vary greatly. Adaptation to chronic stressors leads to a diminished or absent physiological response in persons who have learned to cope with the stressors. Persons who have poor "defense" or coping mechanisms may respond to continuous stress with chronic physiological changes.

In anxiety disorders, the diagnostic subgroups differ on physiological responses quantitatively as well as qualitatively. Moreover, even within a given diagnostic subgroup, physiological response patterns may vary greatly because the diagnostic categories as formulated in DSM-III-R are not homogeneous. Also, constitutional factors and acquired coping mechanisms modify physiological responses.

Patients with chronic anxiety do not appear to be in a constant state of physiological hyperarousal but tend to overreact to situations that are not distressing to normal subjects. Persons with simple phobias overreact only to specific phobic situations. Individuals with social phobias may not constitute a homogeneous group. Some patients may resemble persons with simple phobias, while others may exhibit symptoms of GAD. As expected, persons with social phobias show increased autonomic responses when exposed to feared social situations, but the magnitude of the response is often weak.

Blood-injury phobia takes a special place among phobias because patients with this phobia exhibit a biphasic response to specific stressors that differs from the physiological responses seen in normal subjects and in persons with other anxiety disorders. In blood-injury phobia, the sight of blood or injury induces sympathetic arousal that is followed by a sudden drop in sympathetic tone and possibly a rise in vagal tone. PTSD patients show physiological hyperexcitability to specific, but not to nontraumatic, stimuli. However, because most studies have examined only chronically ill war veterans, it is difficult to generalize to the entire PTSD population.

Increased muscle tension appears to be the prevalent physiological manifestation of chronic anxiety disorders, including GAD, OCD, and panic disorder. Patients with GAD and OCD show little physiological differences during baseline but exhibit diminished autonomic flexibility during laboratory stress. GAD, however, may be a heterogeneous disorder, and subgroups of GAD may differ in their cardiovascular or gastrointestinal reactivity.

Panic disorder has been the most investigated anxiety disorder. Patients with panic disorder exhibit specific physiological responses that are induced by a sudden increase in sympathetic tone, or possibly by a decrease in vagal tone. Some, but not all, panic disorder patients overreact autonomically to relatively innocuous conditions. The tendency to overreact may be associated with the severity of the disorder. While physiological responses to panic attacks are generally mild, physiologically predisposed patients react with dramatic increases in heart rate and blood pressure. Such patients, as well as panic disorder patients who suffer from cardiovascular diseases, may represent a high-risk group for premature death.

The unpredictable responses of stress hormones to subjective anxiety in anxiety disorder patients contrast with the more predictable responses in nonanxious persons. The reason for this discrepancy is unknown and needs further exploration. Studies that use hormonal challenge techniques will most likely provide the answers.

All chronic anxiety disorders exhibit diminished autonomic flexibility and adaptability to stressors. This phenomenon is not disorder specific. It may represent a constitutional autonomic weakness that underlies all chronic anxiety disorders or an inadequate attempt by the body to adapt to chronic anxiety, or it may be due to psychological disregard of nonspecific, but generally stressful, tasks in persons who have narrowed their attention to pathology-related subjects.

There are still many gaps in our understanding of the physiology of anxiety. However, with improved diagnostic and technical tools, and a better understanding of normal and abnormal physiology, our knowledge of peripheral manifestations of anxiety and their interactions with the central nervous system is broadening rapidly.

REFERENCES

American Psychiatric Association: Diagnostic and Statistical Manual of Mental Disorders, 3rd Edition, Revised. Washington, DC, American Psychiatric Association, 1987

Anderson G, Brown RIF: Real and laboratory gambling, sensation-seeking and arousal. Br J Psychology 75:401–410, 1984

Ballenger JC (ed): Toward an integrated model of panic disorder. Am J Orthopsychiatry 59:284–293, 1989

Ballenger JC (ed): Clinical Aspects of Panic Disorder. New York, Wiley, 1990a

Ballenger JC (ed): Neurobiology of Panic Disorder. New York, Wiley, 1990b

Balon R, Ortiz A, Pohl R, et al: Heart rate and blood pressure during placebo-associated panic attacks. Psychosom Med 50:434–438, 1988

Balshan ID: Muscle tension and personality in women. Arch Gen Psychiatry 7:64–76, 1962

Bass C, Kartsounis L, Lelliott P: Hyperventilation and its relationship to anxiety and panic. Integrative Psychiatry 5:274–291, 1987

Beck JG, Scott SK: Physiological and symptom responses to hyperventilation: a comparison of frequent and infrequent panickers. Journal of Psychopathology and Behavior Assessment 10:117–127, 1988

Beech HR, Liddell A: Decision-making, mood states and ritualistic behaviour among obsessional patients, in Obsessional States. Edited by Beech HR. London, Methuen, 1974, pp 143–160

Beidel DC, Turner SM, Dancu CV: Physiological, cognitive, and behavioral aspects of social anxiety. Behaviour Research and Therapy 23:109–117, 1985

Blanchard EB, Kolb LC, Pallmeyer TR, et al: A psychophysiological study of post traumatic stress disorder in Vietnam veterans. Psychiatr Q 54:220–229, 1982

Blanchard EB, Kolb LC, Gerardi RJ, et al: Cardiac response to relevant stimuli as an adjunctive tool for diagnosing post-traumatic stress disorder in Vietnam veterans. Behaviour Research and Therapy 17:592–606, 1986

Boulougouris JC: Variables affecting outcome in obsessive-compulsive patients treated by flooding, in Treatment of Phobic and Obsessive-Compulsive Disorder. Edited by Boulougouris JC, Rabavilas AD. Oxford, UK, Pergamon Press, 1977, pp 73–84

Boulougouris JC, Rabavilas AD, Stefanis C: Psychophysiological responses in obsessive-compulsive patients. Behaviour Research and Therapy 5:221–230, 1977

Bourne PB, Rose RM, Mason JW: 17-OHCS levels in combat: special forces "A" team under threat of attack. Arch Gen Psychiatry 19:135–140, 1968

Brady JP: Social skill training for psychiatric patients, I: concepts, methods and clinical results. Am J Psychiatry 141:333–340, 1984

Breier A: Experimental approaches to human stress research: assessment of neurobiological mechanisms of stress in volunteers and psychiatric patients. Biol Psychiatry 26:438–462, 1989

Burchfield SR: The stress response: a new perspective. Psychosom Med 41:661–672, 1979

Cameron OG, Gunsher S, Hariharan M: Venous plasma epinephrine levels and the symptoms of stress. Psychosom Med 52:411–424, 1990a

Cameron OG, Smith CB, Lee MA, et al: Adrenergic status in anxiety disorders: platelet alpha2-adrenergic receptor binding, blood pressure, pulse, and catecholamines in panic and generalized anxiety disorder patients and in normal subjects. Biol Psychiatry 28:3–20, 1990b

Charney DS, Heninger GR: Abnormal regulation of noradrenergic function in panic disorder. Arch Gen Psychiatry 43:1041–1054, 1986

Charney DS, Heninger GR, Breier A: Noradrenergic function in panic anxiety. Arch Gen Psychiatry 41:751–763, 1984

Charney DS, Heninger GR, Jatlow PI: Increased angiogenic effects of caffeine in panic disorder. Arch Gen Psychiatry 42:233–243, 1985

Charney DS, Woods SW, Goodman WK, et al: Serotonin function in anxiety, II: effects of the serotonin agonist MCPP in panic disorder patients and healthy subjects. Psychopharmacology (Berlin) 92:14–24, 1987

Chosy J, Graham D: Catecholamines in vasovagal fainting. J Psychosom Res 9:189–194, 1965

Clouse RE: Anxiety and gastrointestinal illness. Psychiatr Clin North Am 11:399–417, 1988

Cobb S, Rose RM: Hypertension, peptic ulcer and diabetes in air traffic controllers. JAMA 224:489–492, 1973

Cohen AS, Barlow DH, Blanchard EB: Psychophysiology of relaxation-associated panic attacks. J Abnorm Psychol 94:96–101, 1985

Coryell W, Noyes R, Clancy J: Excess mortality in panic disorder. Arch Gen Psychiatry 39:701–703, 1982

Cowley DS, Hyde TS, Dager SR, et al: Lactate infusion: the role of baseline anxiety. Psychiatry Res 21:169–179, 1987

Craske MG, Sanderson WC, Barlow DH: How do desynchronous response systems relate to the treatment of agoraphobia: a follow-up evaluation. Behaviour and Research Therapy 25:117–122, 1987

Curtis GC, Thyer B: Fainting on exposure to phobic stimuli. Am J Psychiatry 140:771–774, 1983

Curtis GC, Buxton M, Lippman D, et al: "Flooding in vivo" during the circadian phase of minimal cortisol secretion: anxiety and therapeutic success without adrenal cortical activation. Biol Psychiatry 11:101–107, 1976

Curtis GC, Nesse R, Buxton M, et al: Anxiety and plasma cortisol at the crest of the circadian cycle: reappraisal of a classical hypothesis. Psychosom Med 40:368–378, 1978

Curtis GC, Nesse R, Buxton M, et al: Plasma growth hormone: effect of anxiety during flooding in vivo. Am J Psychiatry 136:410–414, 1979

Davidson JRT, Kudler HS, Smith RD: Assessment and pharmacotherapy of posttraumatic stress disorder, in Assessment and Treatment of Posttraumatic Stress Disorder. Edited by Giller EL Jr. Washington, DC, American Psychiatric Press, 1990, pp

Davies AO, Mares A, Pool JL, et al: Mitral valve prolapse with symptoms of beta-adrenergic hypersensitivity. Am J Med 82:193–201, 1987

Dimsdale JE: Generalizing from laboratory studies to field studies of human stress physiology. Psychosom Med 46:463–469, 1984

Dimsdale JE, Moss J: Short-term catecholamine response to psychological stress. Psychosom Med 42:493–497, 1980

Dobbs D, Wilson WP: Observations on persistence of war neurosis. Diseases of the Nervous System 21:686–691, 1960

Eliasson K: Borderline hypertension: circulatory, sympatho-adrenal and psychological reactions to stress. Acta Med Scand Suppl 692:1–90, 1984

Falkner B, Onesti G, Angelakos ET, et al: Cardiovascular response to mental stress in normal adolescents with hypertensive parents. Hypertension 1:23–30, 1979

Fenz WD, Epstein S: Gradients of physiological arousal in parachutists as a function of an approaching jump. Psychosom Med 29:33–51, 1967

Ford MJ: The irritable bowel syndrome. J Psychosom Res 30:399–410, 1986

Forsman L: Habitual catecholamine excretion and its relation to habitual distress. Biol Psychol 11:83–97, 1980

Forsman L, Lindblad LE: Effect of mental stress on baroreceptor-mediated changes in blood pressure and heart rate and on plasma catecholamines and subjective responses in healthy men and women. Psychosom Med 45:435–445, 1983

Frankenhaeuser M: Psychoneuroendocrine approaches to the study of emotion as related to stress and coping. Nebr Symp Motiv, 1979, pp 123–161

Frankenhaeuser M: The sympathetic-adrenal and pituitary-adrenal response to challenge: comparison between the sexes, in Biobehavioral Basis of Coronary Heart Disease. Edited by Dembroski TM, Schmidt TH, Blümchen GS. Basel, S Karger, 1983, pp 91–105

Freedman RR, Ianni P, Ettedgui E, et al: Ambulatory monitoring of panic disorder. Arch Gen Psychiatry 42:244–248, 1985

Fried R: The Hyperventilation Syndrome. Baltimore, MD, Johns Hopkins University Press, 1987

Gaffney FA, Fenton BJ, Lane LD, et al: Hemodynamic, ventilatory, and biochemical responses of panic patients and normal controls with sodium lactate infusion and spontaneous panic attacks. Arch Gen Psychiatry 45:53–60, 1988

Gellhorn E: The neurophysiological basis of anxiety: a hypothesis. Perspect Biol Med 8:488–515, 1965

George DT, Nutt DJ, Walker WV, et al: Lactate and hyperventilation substantially attenuate vagal tone in normal volunteers. Arch Gen Psychiatry 46:153–156, 1989

Giller EL Jr (ed): Biological Assessment and Treatment of Posttraumatic Stress Disorder. Washington, DC, American Psychiatric Press, 1990

Glucksman ML, Quinlan DM, Leigh H: Skin conductance changes and psychotherapeutic content in the treatment of a phobic patient. Br J Med Psychol 58:155–163, 1985

Gorman JM, Fyer AJ, Ross DC, et al: Normalization of venous pH, pCO_2, and bicarbonate levels after blockade of panic attacks. Psychiatry Res 14:57–65, 1985

Gorman JM, Cohen BS, Liebowitz MR, et al: Blood gas changes and hypohasphatemia in lactate-induced panic. Arch Gen Psychiatry 43:1067–1071, 1986

Gorman JM, Fyer MR, Goetz R, et al: Ventilatory physiology of patients with panic disorder. Arch Gen Psychiatry 45:31–39, 1988

Graham DT, Kabler JD, Lunsford L: Vasovagal fainting: a diphasic response. Psychosom Med 23:493–507, 1961

Grillon C, Buchsbaum MS: EEG topography of response to visual stimuli in generalized anxiety disorder. Electroencephalogr Clin Neurophysiol 66:337–348, 1987

Hastrup JL, Light KC, Obrist PA: Paternal hypertension and cardiovascular response to stress in healthy young adults. Psychophysiology 19:615–622, 1982

Heimberg RG, Barlow DH: Psychosocial treatment for social phobia. Psychosomatics 29:27–37, 1988

Hibbert G, Pilsbury D: Hyperventilation: is it a cause of panic attacks? Br J Psychiatry 155:805–809, 1989

Hickey AJ, Andrews G, Wilcken DEL: Independence of mitral valve prolapse and neurosis. Br Heart J 50:333–336, 1983

Hodgson RJ, Rachman S: The effects of contamination and washing in obsessional patients. Behaviour Research and Therapy 10:111–117, 1972

Hoehn-Saric R, Masek BJ: Effects of naloxone in normals and chronically anxious patients. Biol Psychiatry 16:1041–1050, 1981

Hoehn-Saric R, McLeod DR: The peripheral sympathetic nervous system: its role in normal and pathological anxiety. Psychiatr Clin North Am 11:375–386, 1988

Hoehn-Saric R, McLeod DR: Generalized anxiety disorder in adulthood, in Handbook of Child and Adult Psychopathology. Edited by Hersen M, Last CG. New York, Pergamon, 1990, pp 247–260

Hoehn-Saric R, McLeod DR, Zimmerli WD: Subjective and somatic manifestations of anxiety in obsessive-compulsive and generalized anxiety disorder. Paper presented at the 141st annual meeting of the American Psychiatric Association, Montreal, May 1988

Hoehn-Saric R, McLeod DR, Zimmerli WD: Somatic manifestations in women with generalized anxiety disorder: physiological responses to psychological stress. Arch Gen Psychiatry 46:1113–1119, 1989a

Hoehn-Saric R, McLeod DR, Zimmerli WD: Symptoms and treatment response to generalized anxiety disorder patients with high versus low levels of cardiovascular complaints. Am J Psychiatry 146:854–859, 1989b

Hoehn-Saric R, McLeod DR, Lee YB, et al: Cortisol levels in generalized anxiety disorder (letter). Psychiatry Res 38:313–315, 1991a

Hoehn-Saric R, McLeod DR, Zimmerli WD: Psychophysiological response patterns in panic disorder. Acta Psychiatr Scand 83:4–11, 1991b

Holden AE Jr, Barlow DH: Heart rate and heart rate variability recorded in vivo in agoraphobics and nonphobics. Behavior Therapy 17:26–42, 1986

Holt PE, Andrews G: Hyperventilation and anxiety in panic disorder, social phobia, GAD and normal controls. Behaviour Research and Therapy 27:453–460, 1989

Insel TR, Zahn T, Murphy DL: Obsessive-compulsive disorder: an anxiety disorder? in Anxiety and the Anxiety Disorders. Edited by Tuma AT, Maser J. Hillsdale, NJ, Lawrence Erlbaum, 1985, pp 577–589

Jacob RG: Panic disorder and vestibular system. Psychiatr Clin North Am 11:361–374, 1988

James W: The Principles of Psychology. New York, Holt, Rinehart and Winston, 1890

Jenike MA, Bear L, Minichiello WE: Obsessive-Compulsive Disorders: Theory and Management, 2nd Edition. Chicago, IL, Year Book Medical Publishers, 1990

Johansson J, Öst LG: Perception of autonomic reactions and actual heart rate in phobic patients. Journal of Behavioral Assessment 4:133–143, 1982

Jonsson A, Hanssen L: Prolonged exposure to a stressful stimulus (noise) as a cause of raised blood pressure in man. Lancet 1:86–87, 1977

Kagan J, Reznik JS, Snidman N: Biological basis of childhood shyness. Science 240:167–171, 1988

Kasvikis YG, Basoglu M, Monteiro W, et al: Urinary cortisol during exposure in obsessive-compulsive ritualizers. Psychiatry Res 23:131–135, 1988

Kathol RG, Noyes R Jr, Lopez AL, et al: Relationship of urinary free cortisol levels in patients with panic disorder to symptoms of depression and agoraphobia. Psychiatry Res 24:211–221, 1988

Kelly D: Anxiety and Emotions. Springfield, IL, Charles C Thomas, 1980

Kirschbaum C, Hellhammer DH: Salivary cortisol in psychobiological research: an overview. Neuropsychobiology 22:150–169, 1989

Ko GN, Elsworth JD, Ruth RH, et al: Panic-induced elevation of plasma MHPG levels in phobic-anxious patients. Arch Gen Psychiatry 40:425–450, 1983

Kosten TR, Mason JW, Giller EL, et al: Sustained urinary norepinephrine and epinephrine elevation in post-traumatic stress disorder. Psycho-endocrinology 12:13–20, 1987

Kunin CM, McCormack RC: Epidemiologic study of bacteriuria and blood pressure among nuns and working women. N Engl J Med 278:635–642, 1968

Lader MH: Palmar conductance measures in anxiety and phobic states. J Psychosom Res 11:271–281, 1967

Lader MH, Mathews A: Physiological changes during spontaneous panic attacks. J Psychosom Res 14:377–382, 1970

Lader MH, Wing L: Habituation of the psycho-galvanic reflex in patients with anxiety states and in normal subjects. J Neurol Neurosurg Psychiatry 27:210–218, 1964

Lader MH, Gelder MG, Marks IM: Palmar skin-conductance measures as predictors of response to desensitization. J Psychosom Res 11:283–290, 1967

Lande SD: Physiological and subjective measures of anxiety during flooding. Behaviour Research and Therapy 20:472–490, 1982

Lelliott PT, Noshirvani HF, Marks IM, et al: Relationship of skin-conductance activity to clinical features in obsessive-compulsive ritualizers. Psychol Med 17:905–914, 1987

Levi L: The urinary output of adrenaline and noradrenaline during pleasant and unpleasant emotional states. Psychosom Med 27:80–85, 1965

Levin AP, Doran AR, Liebowitz MR, et al: Pituitary adrenal unresponsiveness in lactate-induced panic. Psychiatry Res 21:23–32, 1987

Ley R: Agoraphobia, the panic attack and the hyperventilation syndrome. Behaviour Research and Therapy 23:79–81, 1985

Liebowitz MR, Gorman JM, Fyer AJ, et al: Lactate provocation of panic attacks, II: biochemical and physiological findings. Arch Gen Psychiatry 42:709–719, 1985a

Liebowitz MR, Gorman JM, Fyer AJ, et al: Social phobia: review of a neglected anxiety disorder. Arch Gen Psychiatry 42:729–736, 1985b

Lovallo WR, Pincomb GA, Brackett DJ, et al: Heart rate reactivity as a predictor of neuroendocrine responses to aversive and appetitive challenges. Psychosom Med 52:17–26, 1990

Lum LC: Hyperventilation: the tip of the iceberg. J Psychosom Res 19:375–383, 1975

Malloy PF, Fairbank JA, Keane TM: Validation of a multimethod assessment of posttraumatic stress disorder in Vietnam veterans. J Consult Clin Psychol 51:488–494, 1983

Malmo RB: Anxiety and behavioral arousal. Psychol Res 64:276–287, 1957

Malmo RB, Smith AA, Kohlmeyer WA: Motor manifestations of conflict in interviews: a case study. Journal of Abnormal and Social Psychology 52:268–271, 1956

Marks IM: Fears, Phobias, and Rituals. New York, Oxford University Press, 1987

Marks IM: Blood-injury phobia: a review. Am J Psychiatry 145:1207–1213, 1988

Mason JW, Giller EL, Kosten TR, et al: Urinary free cortisol levels in posttraumatic stress disorder patients. J Nerv Ment Dis 174:145–149, 1986

Mason JW, Giller EL, Kosten TR, et al: Elevation of urinary norepinephrine/cortisol ratio in posttraumatic stress disorder. J Nerv Ment Dis 176:498–502, 1988

Mathew RJ, Ho BT, Kralik P, et al: Catecholamines and monoamine oxidase activity in anxiety. Acta Psychiatr Scand 63:245–252, 1981

Mathew RJ, Ho BT, Frances DJ, et al: Catecholamines and anxiety. Acta Psychiatr Scand 65:142–147, 1982

Mathews AM: Psychophysiological approaches to the investigation of desensitization and related procedures. Psychol Bull 76:73–91, 1971

Mavissakalian M, Michelson L: Patterns of psychophysiological change in the treatment of agoraphobia. Behaviour and Research Therapy 20:347–356, 1982

McCance AJ: Assessment of sympathoneural activity in clinical research. Life Sci 48:713–721, 1991

McFall ME, Murburg MM, Ko GN, et al: Autonomic responses to stress in Vietnam combat veterans with posttraumatic stress disorder. Biol Psychiatry 27:1165–1175, 1990

McFarlane AC: The aetiology of post-traumatic stress disorders following a natural disaster. Br J Psychiatry 152:116–121, 1988

Menzies DN: Vasovagal shock after insertion of intrauterine device. BMJ 1:305, 1978

Merckelbach H, van Hout W, van den Hout MA, et al: Psychophysiological and subjective reactions of social phobics and normals to facial stimuli. Behaviour Research and Therapy 27:289–294, 1989

Munjack DJ, Baltazar PL, De Quattro V, et al: Generalized anxiety disorder: some biochemical aspects. Psychiatry Res 32:35–43, 1990

Murburg MM, McFall ME, Veith RC: Catecholamines, stress, and post-traumatic stress disorder, in Biological Assessment and Treatment of Posttraumatic Stress Disorder. Edited by Giller EL Jr. Washington, DC, American Psychiatric Press, 1990, pp

Nesse RM, Curtis GC, Brown GM, et al: Anxiety induced by flooding therapy for phobias does not elicit prolactin secretion response. Psychosom Med 42:25–31, 1980

Nesse RM, Curtis GC, Thyer BA, et al: Endocrine and cardiovascular responses during phobic anxiety. Psychosom Med 47:320–332, 1985

Odio MR, Brodish A: Effects of chronic stress on in vivo pituitary adrenocortical responses to corticotropin-releasing hormone. Neuropeptides 15:143–152, 1990

Orr SP: Psychophysiologic studies of posttraumatic stress disorder, in Biological Assessment of Posttraumatic Stress Disorder. Edited by Giller EL Jr. Washington, DC, American Psychiatric Press, 1990, pp 135–137

Öst LG, Jerremalm A, Johansson J: Individual response patterns and the effects of different behavioral methods in the treatment of social phobia. Behaviour Research and Therapy 19:1–16, 1981

Öst LG, Sterner V, Lindahl I: Physiological responses in blood phobics. Behaviour Research and Therapy 22:109–117, 1984

Pallmeyer TP, Blanchard EB, Kolb LC: The psychophysiology of combat-induced post-traumatic stress disorder in Vietnam veterans. Behaviour Research and Therapy 24:645–652, 1986

Papp LA, Martinez J, Gorman JM: Arterial epinephrine levels in panic disorder. Psychiatry Res 25:111–112, 1988

Peronnet F, Blier P, Brisson G, et al: Plasma catecholamines at rest and exercise in subjects with high- and low-trait anxiety. Psychosom Med 48:52–58, 1986

Pincus JH, Tucker GJ: Behavioral Neurology, 3rd Edition. New York, Oxford University Press, 1985

Pitman RK, Orr SP, Forgue DF, et al: Psychophysiologic assessment of posttraumatic stress disorder imagery in Vietnam combat veterans. Arch Gen Psychiatry 44:970–975, 1987

Pohl R, Ettedgui E, Bridges M, et al: Plasma MHPG levels in lactate and isoproterenol anxiety states. Biol Psychiatry 22:1127–1136, 1987

Porges SW: Respiratory sinus arrhythmia: physiological basis, quantitative methods, and clinical implication, in Cardiorespiratory and Cardiosomatic Psychophysiology. Edited by Grossman P, Janssen KHL, Vaitl D. New York, Plenum, 1986, pp 101–115

Rachman S, Hodgson RJ: Synchrony and desynchrony in fear and avoidance. Behaviour Research and Therapy 12:311–318, 1974

Rachman SJ, Hodgson RJ: Obsessions and Compulsions. Englewood Cliffs, NJ, Prentice-Hall, 1980

Rapaport MH, Risch SC, Golshan S, et al: Neuroendocrine effects of ovine corticotropin-releasing hormone in panic disorder patients. Biol Psychiatry 26:344–348, 1989

Roessler R: Personality, psychophysiology, and performance. Psychophysiology 10:315–327, 1973

Rose RM: Overview of endocrinology of stress, in Neuroendocrinology and Psychiatric Disorders. Edited by Brown GM, Koslow SH, Reichlin S. New York, Raven, 1984, pp 95–112

Rose RM, Chesney MA: Cardiovascular stress reactivity: a behavior-genetic perspective. Behaviour Research and Therapy 17:314–324, 1986

Rosenbaum AH, Schatzberg AF, Jost FA, et al: Urinary free cortisol levels in anxiety. Psychosomatics 24:835–837, 1983

Roth WT, Telch MJ, Taylor CB, et al: Autonomic characteristics of agoraphobia with panic attacks. Biol Psychiatry 21:1133–1154, 1986

Roth WT, Ehlers A, Taylor CB et al: Skin conductance habituation in panic disorder patients. Biol Psychiatry 27:1231–1243, 1990

Rotter JB: Generalized Expectancies for Internal vs External Control of Reinforcement. Psychological Monographs, Vol 80, No 1, 1966

Rozanski A, Bairey N, Krantz DS, et al: Mental stress and the indication of silent myocardial ischemia in patients with coronary artery disease. N Engl J Med 318:1005–1012, 1988

Ruetz PP, Johnson SA, Callahan R, et al: Fainting: a review of its mechanisms and a study in blood donors. Medicine 46:363–383, 1967

Schaeffer MA, Baum A: Adrenal cortical response to stress at Three Mile Island. Psychosom Med 46:227–237, 1984

Schnall PL, Pieper C, Schwartz JE, et al: The relationship between "job strain," workplace diastolic blood pressure, and left ventricular mass index. JAMA 263:1929–1935, 1990

Schneider P, Evans L, Ross-Lee L, et al: Plasma biogenic amine levels in agoraphobia with panic attacks. Pharmacopsychiatry 20:102–104, 1987

Schneier FR, Liebowitz MR: Social phobia in adulthood, in Handbook of Child and Adult Psychopathology. Edited by Hersen M, Last CG. New York, Pergamon, 1990, pp 169–180

Sevy S, Papadimitriou GN, Surmont DW, et al: Noradrenergic function in generalized anxiety disorder, major depression disorder, and healthy subjects. Biol Psychiatry 25:141–152, 1989

Shapiro D, Crider A: Psychophysiological approaches in social psychology, in the Handbook of Social Psychology, 2nd Edition, Vol 3. Edited by Lindzey G, Aronson E. Addison-Wesley, 1969

Shear MK: Pathophysiology of panic: a review of pharmacological tests and naturalistic monitoring data. J Clin Psychiatry 47 (suppl 6):18–26, 1986

Shear MK, Kligfield P, Harshfield G, et al: Cardiac rate and rhythm in panic patients. Am J Psychiatry 144:633–638, 1987

Starkman MN, Zelnik TC, Nesse RM, et al: Anxiety in patients with pheochromocytoma. Arch Intern Med 145:248–252, 1985

Steptoe A: Stress, helplessness and control: the implications of laboratory studies. J Psychosom Res 27:361–367, 1983

Steptoe A: The assessment of sympathetic nervous function in human stress research. J Psychosom Res 31:141–152, 1987

Steptoe A, Wardle J: Emotional fainting and the psychophysiologic response to blood and injury: autonomic mechanisms and coping strategies. Psychosom Med 50:402–417, 1988

Taylor CB, Telch MJ, Havvik D: Ambulatory heart rate changes during panic attacks. J Psychiat Res 17:261–266, 1983

Taylor CB, Sheikh J, Agras WS, et al: Ambulatory heart rate changes in patients with panic attacks. Am J Psychiatry 143:478–482, 1986

Taylor CB, King R, Ehlers A, et al: Treadmill exercise test and ambulatory measures in panic attacks. Am J Cardiol 60:48J–52J, 1987

Tecce JJ: Contingent negative variation (CNV) and psychological processes in man. Psychol Bull 77:73–108, 1972

Thakor NV, Yang M, Amaresan M, et al: A microcomputer-based ambulatory monitor for vital signs in anxiety disorders. Journal of Ambulatory Monitoring 2:277–294, 1989

Thyer BA, Himle J, Curtis GC: Blood-injury illness phobia: a review. J Clin Psychol 41:451–459, 1985

Turner SM, Beidel DC, Dancu CV, et al: Psychopathology of social phobia and comparison to avoidant personality disorder. J Abnorm Psychol 95:389–394, 1986

Uhde TW, Boulenger JP, Roy-Byrne PP, et al: Longitudinal course of panic disorder: clinical and biological considerations. Prog Neuropsychopharmacol Biol Psychiatry 9:39–51, 1985

Uhde TW, Joffe RT, Jimerson DC, et al: Normal urinary free cortisol and plasma MHPG in panic disorder: clinical and theoretical implications. Biol Psychiatry 23:575–585, 1988

Ursin H, Baade E, Levine S: Psychobiology of Stress. New York, Academic, 1978

Villacres EC, Hollifield M, Katon WJ, et al: Sympathetic nervous system activity in panic disorder. Psychiatry Res 21:313–321, 1987

Wallin G, Sundlöf G: Sympathetic outflow of muscles during vasovagal syncope. J Auton Nerv Syst 6:287–291, 1982

Weiner H: The psychobiology and pathophysiology of anxiety and fear, in Anxiety and Anxiety Disorders. Edited by Tuma AH, Maser J. Hillside, NJ, Lawrence Erlbaum, 1985, pp 333–354

Weissman MM: The epidemiology of anxiety disorder, in Anxiety and Anxiety Disorders. Edited by Tuma AH, Maser J. Hillside, NJ, Lawrence Erlbaum, 1985, pp 275–296

Weissman NJ, Shear MK, Kramer-Fox R, et al: Contrasting patterns of autonomic dysfunction in patients with mitral valve prolapse and panic attacks. Am J Med 82:880–888, 1987

Weissman MM, Markowitz JS, Ovelette R, et al: Panic disorder and cardiovascular/cerebrovascular problems: results from a community survey. Am J Psychiatry 147:1504–1508, 1990

Williams RB Jr, Lane D, Kuhn CM, et al: Type A behavior and elevated physiological and neuroendocrine responses to cognitive tasks. Science 218:483–485, 1982

Wolf ME, Mosnaim AD (eds): Posttraumatic Stress Disorder: Etiology, Phenomenology, and Treatment. Washington, DC, American Psychiatric Press, 1990

Woods SW, Charney DS, McPherson CA, et al: Situational panic attacks. Arch Gen Psychiatry 44:365–375, 1987

Woods SW, Charney DS, Goodman WK, et al: Carbon dioxide–induced anxiety. Arch Gen Psychiatry 45:43–52, 1988

Yaragani VK, Balon R, Pohl R: Lactate infusion in panic disorder patients and normal controls: autonomic measures and subjective anxiety. Acta Psychiatr Scand 79:32–40, 1989

Yaragani VK, Balon R, Pohl R, et al: Decreased R-R variance in panic disorder patients. Acta Psychiatr Scand 81:554–559, 1990a

Yaragani VK, Meiri PC, Pohl R, et al: Heart rate and blood pressure changes during postural changes and isometric handgrip exercise in patients with panic disorder and normal controls. Acta Psychiatr Scand 81:9–13, 1990b

Yaragani VK, Pohl R, Balon R, et al: Heartrate in panic disorder. Acta Psychiatr Scand 83:79, 1991

Yehuda R, Southwick SM, Nussbaum G, et al: Low urinary cortisol excretion in patients with posttraumatic stress disorder. J Nerv Ment Dis 178:366–369, 1990

Chapter 6

Perception of Physiological Changes in Normal and Pathological Anxiety

Daniel R. McLeod, Ph.D., and
Rudolf Hoehn-Saric, M.D.

For both clinical and theoretical reasons it is important to know how well patients with anxiety disorders can perceive bodily changes. For example, the choice of treatment regimens is often determined on the basis of somatic symptom reports. In this chapter we will examine what is known about the relationship between somatic symptom reports and their underlying physiological referents.

ACCURACY OF SOMATIC SYMPTOM REPORTS

When patients with anxiety complain of increased sweating or heart palpitations, should we believe them? The literature on self-report suggests that perhaps we should not. After all, many studies have demonstrated poor correlations between somatic symptom reports and their physiological referents (Pennebaker 1982; Ray et al. 1983). And yet, one needs only to shake the hand of an anxious patient who complains of sweaty palms to realize that, at least on some occasions, patients' self-reports are correct. How can this apparent contradiction be resolved? The answer to this question requires an assessment of the accuracy of somatic symptom reports.

By the term *symptom* we mean the patient's subjective perception of a physiological state or activity. By the term *accuracy* we mean the correspondence between a given physiological state or activity and the perception of that state or activity (Pennebaker 1982). In the pages that follow, we will be discussing only the relationships between physiological states or activities and verbal reports of these states or activities. Discussions of more global concepts such as mood or arousal can be found elsewhere in the literature (MacKay 1980; Skelton and Pennebaker 1990; Zillmann 1983).

Knowledge of the accuracy of patient symptom reports is important for several reasons. It is important clinically because we often need to know that what patients tell us is actually the case prior to initiating certain treatment regimens. Several studies have shown that patients with chronic diseases tend to rely more on symptoms than on objective measures to monitor their conditions (Skelton and Pennebaker 1990). It is important from a theoretical perspective because we often wish to test hypotheses about the effects of various treatments, etiology of a disorder, and so forth. For example, we may wish to know whether or not an increase in heart rate is reacted to catastrophically by patients with panic disorder (Beck and Emery 1985; Clark 1986). This can be true only if patients can detect changes in heart rate. And patients with anxiety present a special problem because their symptom reports are exaggerated compared with those of nonanxious populations (Hoehn-Saric et al. 1989).

SYMPTOM PERCEPTION AND ANXIETY

Persons with high levels of anxiety tend to report more somatic symptoms than do nonanxious persons (Pennebaker 1982), but are their symptom perceptions more accurate? A study by Schandry (1981) found that subjects who scored higher on state anxiety, as measured by the STATE form of the State-Trait Anxiety Inventory (Spielberger et al. 1970), were more accurate than those with lower anxiety scores on a heartbeat detection task. However, subsequent studies by Montgomery and Jones (1984) and by Weisz et al. (1988) failed to replicate these findings using more sophisticated heartbeat detection tasks.

Several studies have reported that accuracy in visceral perception is greater under conditions of heightened physiological arousal (Katkin 1985; Montgomery et al. 1984; Schandry and

Specht 1981). It is possible that during periods of intense anxiety, patients become more highly aroused physiologically and thus become more accurate at perceiving physiological activity. Unfortunately, none of the above studies used patients with clinical levels of anxiety as subjects. Under relatively nonstressful conditions, patients with generalized anxiety disorder (GAD) tend to exhibit elevated muscle tension but not elevated heart rate, skin conductance, or respiration frequency (Hoehn-Saric et al. 1989). Under stress, these activities do increase, but the one study to date that has assessed symptom reports in clinically anxious patients under stress (McLeod et al. 1986) failed to find increased accuracy. This may, however, have been due to the fact that the degree of stress produced in the latter study was not great. Future studies involving greater levels of stress would be helpful in this regard. On the other hand, several studies have found elevated heart rates and blood pressure in panic disorder patients who have frequent panic attacks (see Hoehn-Saric and McLeod, Chapter 5, this volume; McLeod and Hoehn-Saric 1990). And yet, Ehlers et al. (1988) have found that patients with panic disorder are no more accurate than normal control subjects in perceiving their heart rates.

Other studies have examined the relationship between self-reported levels of anxiety and measurements of physiological activity. For example, Morrow and Labrum (1978) compared several anxiety rating scales with physiological measures, Scott and Kessler (1969) compared subject-reported levels of anxiety with skin conductance, and Tyrer and Lader (1976) compared subject-reported levels of anxiety with heart rate, respiration rate, skin conductance level, and skin conductance fluctuations. These studies and most others have found poor correlations between levels of self-reported anxiety and physiological states. One exception is a study by Thyer et al. (1984). These investigators found positive within-subject correlations between heart rate and analog ratings of anxiety for some subjects but not for other subjects.

Another series of studies have examined the relationship between physiological states and patient reports of those states. From these studies we can gather information on the accuracy of physiological perception in patients with anxiety disorders.

Tyrer et al. (1980) compared measured heart rate with analog estimates of heart rate in patients with hypochondriasis and patients with chronic anxiety. Whereas the hypochondriacal group showed a fairly good correlation ($r = .50$) between self-reported and actual heart rate, the chronically anxious group (i.e., the anxiety patients) did not ($r = .29$). In a study with panic disorder patients, Ehlers et al. (1988) found that in the absence of training, heartbeat perception accuracy was poor, both in panic disorder patients and in nonanxious volunteers. Interestingly, feedback training improved accuracy in the control group but not in the patients with panic disorder. In another study with panic disorder patients, Pyke and Greenberg (1986) found that norepinephrine infusion produced reports of racing heart and palpitations that were not confirmed by measures of heart rate and cardiac rhythm.

CORRELATIONS BETWEEN SYMPTOM REPORTS AND PHYSIOLOGY

About a decade ago, Pennebaker (1982) examined the correlations between symptom reports and their physiological referents obtained from a number of his own studies, using both within- and between-subject methodologies, and found the correlations to be quite low. This has tended to be the case in more recent studies as well (Ehlers et al. 1988; Katkin 1985). Accuracy of physiological perception varies widely across studies but tends, in general, to be quite low when correlational analyses are used. Does this mean that when patients report increases in heart rate, muscle tension, or sweating, they will be correct only at the level of chance?

A few years back we (McLeod et al. 1986) did a study of patients with GAD in which we examined the effects of an automated version of the Stroop test (Stroop 1935) on two sets of measures: 1) physiological measures, consisting of heart interbeat interval (the reciprocal of heart rate), skin conductance, frontalis electromyographic activity, and gastrocnemius electromyographic activity; and 2) analog subject ratings of heart palpitations, sweating, shaking/trembling, and muscle tension. In the automated Stroop test, the words "red," "green," and "blue" are presented on a video screen in block letters colored in red, green, or blue. For example, the word "red" might be presented in blue letters, the word "blue" might be presented in green letters, and so forth. The patients were required to press a key associated with the color of the letters, not with the color spelled out by the letters.

Figure 6–1 shows what we found. The top panel presents subject ratings of sweating, heart palpitations, muscle tension, and shaking/trembling during baseline rest periods (the light histograms) and during the Stroop test (the dark histograms). The bottom panel shows the physiological recordings. Notice that in spite of the fact that the correlations between analog ratings and physiological measures were low, the two sets of measures changed in the same direction during the task: ratings of sweating and skin conductance increased, as did heart palpitations ratings and heart rate (i.e., heart interbeat interval decreased). Ratings of muscle tension and electromyographic activity also tended to increase together.

These data indicate that patient symptom reports can accurately reflect the direction, but not necessarily the degree, of change in physiological activity produced by a stressful task. The low correlation between the two sets of measures simply reflects a quantitative inaccuracy, not a qualitative one. For example, those patients who reported the highest levels of sweatiness were not necessarily the ones who actually did the most sweating. However, reports of increased sweating did correspond with increased skin conductance. This means that, at least under some conditions, a patient who complains of a rapid heart rate probably has a rapid heart rate.

The results of this study are consistent with those of some studies that have compared levels of anxiety, rather than symptom reports, with physiological measures. For example, Sartory et al. (1977) found increases in heart rate with increases in levels of subjective fear in phobic patients. Knight and Borden (1979) found parallel increases in subjective ratings of nervousness and measures of skin conductance and heart rate in socially anxious subjects. In addition, Stern and Marks (1973) found parallel changes in subjective anxiety and heart rate in phobic patients exposed to flooding.

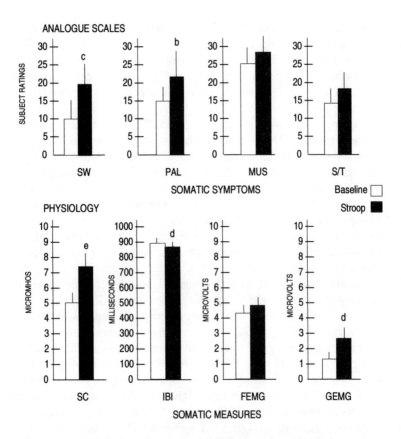

Figure 6–1. Effects of stress on somatic symptoms of anxiety.
(Top) Analog rating scales. *(Bottom)* Physiological measures. X axis:
somatic symptoms and measures. Y axis: subject ratings and
physiological recordings. Lines above the histograms represent
standard errors of the means (SEM). Abbreviations: SW, sweating;
PAL, palpitations; MUS, muscular tension; S/T, shaking/trembling;
SC, mean skin conductance level; IBI, mean heart interbeat interval;
FEMG, frontalis electromyographic activity; GEMG, gastrocnemius
electromyographic activity. Significance levels: b, $P < .05$; c, $P < .02$;
d, $P < .01$; e, $P < .001$. Reprinted by permission of Elsevier Science
Publishing Company, Inc. from"Somatic Symptoms of Anxiety:
Comparison of Self-Report and Physiological Measures, by McLeod
DR, Hoehn-Saric R, Stefan RL. *Biological Psychiatry* 21:301–310, 1986.
Copyright 1986 by the Society of Biological Psychiatry.

CORRELATIONAL VERSUS CATEGORICAL ANALYSIS

The apparent contradiction between the low correlations found in many studies between self-reports and physiological measures and the results of the studies described above, in which patients appeared to correctly report physiological changes, can perhaps be resolved by drawing a distinction between correlational analysis and categorical analysis. In a correlational analysis, a significant finding means that patients showing large increases in, for example, reports of sweating will show large increases in skin conductance. In a categorical analysis, a significant finding means that patients showing any increase in reports of sweating will show at least some increase in skin conductance. In the past, studies have reported low accuracy on the basis of low correlations between symptom reports and their physiological referents. But if the question is a categorical one, such as "Do you sweat more under stress?" then a correlational analysis can be misleading. Patients do tend to sweat more under certain conditions and they know it! The same is true for heart rate perception. Sharpley and Fleming (1988) examined direction and magnitude of subject-estimated heart rate changes in students exposed to a mental arithmetic task that reliably increased heart rate. Of 35 subjects, 13 could not detect heart rate changes, but the other 22 correctly reported the direction, but not the magnitude, of heart rate changes during the task.

Another series of studies that have reported direction of change instead of correlations is that of ambulatory heart rate monitoring in patients with panic disorder. In these studies, the proportion of naturally occurring panic attacks that were accompanied by actual increases in heart rate can provide a measure of accuracy of heart rate perception. Taylor et al. (1983) reported that 3 out of 8 panic attacks were accompanied by elevated heart rates. Gaffney et al. (1988) reported elevated heart rates in 14 out of 31 panic attacks, and Taylor et al. (1986) reported heart rate elevation in 19 out of 33 panic attacks. In addition, Freedman et al. (1985) reported heart rate elevation in 7 out of 8 panic attacks. Thus, the percentages of panic attacks accompanied by increases in heart rate ranged from 38% to 88%. In addition, Margraf et al.

(1987) used an ambulatory monitor to compare spontaneous panic attacks with situational panic attacks and found that heart rate did not change during spontaneous attacks and showed only mild elevations before and during situational attacks. At the present time, too few studies have been conducted for us to know the conditions under which panic attacks will and will not be accompanied by elevated heart rates.

DESYNCHRONY

As we have seen, there are conditions under which patients with anxiety disorders under stress can accurately perceive the direction of change in physiological activities. However, such parallel changes in subjective and physiological measures do not always take place. In a more recent study (McLeod et al. 1990) we examined the subjective and physiological changes in patients with GAD who were treated for 6 weeks with therapeutic doses of either alprazolam or imipramine. In addition to the physiological measures of heart rate, systolic blood pressure, frontalis electromyographic activity, and gastrocnemius electromyographic activity, both investigator and patient reports of cardiovascular and muscular symptoms were obtained before and after 6 weeks of treatment with medication. The investigator-rated scales included the cardiovascular and somatic muscular subscales of the Hamilton Scale of Anxiety (Hamilton 1959). The patient-rated scales included the muscular and cardiopulmonary subscales of the Somatic Symptoms Scale (Hoehn-Saric 1981).

The changes in both somatic symptom reports and physiology following 6 weeks of medication are shown in Figure 6–2. While the changes in physiology following alprazolam are consistent with the changes in symptom reports, the same cannot be said for the effects of imipramine. As is shown in Figure 6–2, decreases in cardiovascular and muscular symptom ratings were accompanied by increases in heart rate, systolic blood pressure, and electromyographic activity. That is, the somatic symptom reports changed in a direction opposite that of their physiological referents following treatment with imipramine.

Similar counterintuitive findings have been reported in studies comparing subjective ratings of anxiety with physiological

changes following treatment. Barlow et al. (1980) reported discrepancies between heart rate and self-reports of anxiety in agoraphobic patients treated with behavioral methods, and
subsequent studies have confirmed these findings. Mavissakalian and Michelson (1982) treated agoraphobic patients for 12

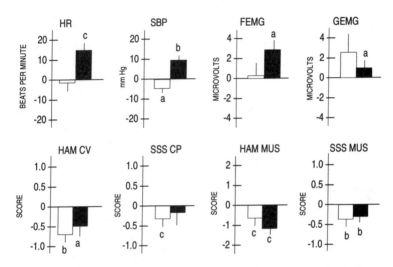

Figure 6–2. Comparison of the effects of treatment on physiological
measures *(top panels)* and somatic symptom reports *(bottom panels)*. All
scores represent mean change (±1 SE) from Week 0 to Week 6
following treatment with alprazolam *(light histograms)* or imipramine
(dark histograms). Abbreviations: HR: heart rate; SBP: systolic blood
pressure; FEMG: frontalis electromyographic activity; GEMG:
gastrocnemius electromyographic activity; HAM CV: Hamilton Scale
of Anxiety, cardiovascular subscale; SSS CP: Somatic Symptoms Scale,
cardiopulmonary subscale; HAM MUS: Hamilton Scale of Anxiety,
muscular subscale; SSS MUS: Somatic Symptoms Scale, muscular
subscale. a: Week 0 and Week 6 values differ ($P < .05$); b: Week 0 and
Week 6 values differ ($P < .01$); c: Week 0 and Week 6 values differ
($P < .001$). Reprinted by permission of Elsevier Science Publishing
Company, Inc. from "Treatment Effects of Alprazolam and
Imipramine: Physiological Versus Subjective Changes in Patients With
Generalized Anxiety Disorder," by McLeod DR, Hoehn-Saric R,
Zimmerli WD, et al. *Biological Psychiatry* 28:849–861, 1990. Copyright
1990 by the Society of Biological Psychiatry.

weeks and noticed frequent discrepancies between changes in heart rate and changes in levels of anxiety. Similar findings were reported by Vermilyea et al. (1984), who compared patient anxiety levels with heart rate over 12 weeks of treatment for agoraphobia. Finally, Roth et al. (1988) found decreases in anxiety levels but increases in heart rate following 15 weeks of treatment with imipramine in agoraphobic patients. These findings are examples of what Rachman and Hodgson (1974) have referred to as "desynchrony." Two sets of measures are said to be desynchronous if they vary independently or inversely from one point in time to another. Grey et al. (1979) have shown that whether changes in heart rate and subjective fear ratings are synchronous or desynchronous may depend upon how demanding the treatment condition is.

PERCEPTION VERSUS DETECTION

How do we explain the fact that somatic symptoms and their physiological referents exhibit synchrony in one context but desynchrony in another? The answer requires a distinction between the processes of perception and detection (Pennebaker and Hoover 1984). In the *detection* of a physiological state the patient uses only physiological information—all other factors are excluded. In the *perception* of a physiological state the patient uses information from a variety of sources. While it is possible that subjects in controlled laboratory settings can detect their heartbeats at a somewhat better-than-chance level (Brener and Kluvitse 1988), the symptom reports of patients with anxiety rarely occur under controlled laboratory conditions. Moreover, symptom reports reflect global sensations, such as rapid heart rate or palpitations, rather than the specific yes-no–type responses obtained in heartbeat detection studies (e.g., Whitehead et al. 1977). These reasons, combined with the observation that patients with anxiety do tend to use information from a variety of sources in reporting somatic symptoms, suggest that somatic symptom reports reflect perception, not detection. (For a good review of visceral detection studies, see Reed et al. 1990.)

Accuracy in the perception of a physiological state depends on many factors other than just the physiological state itself. For example, in a study comparing actual with perceived heart rate during a number of laboratory tasks, Pennebaker and Hoover (1984) found a much stronger correlation between self-reported heart rate and perceived pleasantness of the task ($r = -.74$) than between self-reported and actual heart rate ($r = .36$). Pennebaker and Epstein (1983) have estimated that only about 6% of the variance in symptom reports can be accounted for by the actual physiological state or activity itself.

MECHANISMS OF SYMPTOM PERCEPTION

We can now return to the problem of desynchrony found in the study comparing alprazolam and imipramine (see the section on desynchrony above; see also McLeod et al. 1990). Why would patients report reductions in cardiovascular symptoms when in reality their heart rates and their blood pressures were both increased as a result of 6 weeks of treatment with imipramine? The answer may be that we are dealing in this context not with detection but with perception. If this is so, then we must look to factors other than our physiological measures themselves for an explanation.

Three hypotheses that are at least partially consistent with the results of the alprazolam/imipramine study are as follows:

1. The *variability hypothesis,* which states that change in a physiological state, rather than absolute level, can be used to perceive that state
2. The *attention hypothesis,* which states that awareness of physiological states increases with increased self-attention
3. The *expectation hypothesis,* which states that a person's beliefs about how physiological processes should react in certain circumstances can determine that person's perception of those physiological processes

Variability

As Pennebaker and Skelton (1981) discovered (also see Pennebaker 1982), people can use change in a physiological state, rather than static levels, to perceive that state. One possibility, then, is that patients in the alprazolam/imipramine study were interpreting changes in heart rate or electromyographic activity as elevated heart rate or muscle tension. If this is true, then patients may have reported decreases in somatic symptoms because the variability in the physiological referents of those symptoms decreased with treatment. We have elsewhere referred to this explanation as the "variability" hypothesis (McLeod et al. 1990), and it has two variants. Decreases in the variability of physiological activities could reflect a direct pharmacological effect of medication (*direct variability hypothesis*) or an indirect effect of some other factor, such as fewer episodes of increased anxiety following treatment (*indirect variability hypothesis*).

The effects of pharmacological treatment on heart rate variability are shown in Figures 6–3 and 6–4.

In Figure 6–3, heart rate variability is expressed in terms of the *mean square successive difference* statistic, or MSSD (Heslegrave et

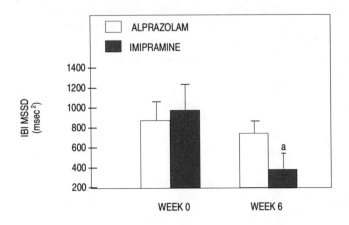

Figure 6–3. Six-week effects of alprazolam *(light histograms)* and imipramine *(dark histograms)* on heart interbeat interval (IBI) variance, represented by the mean square successive difference (MSSD). a: Week 0 and Week 6 values differ ($P < .001$). Values represent the mean ± 1 SE. Reprinted, by permission of Elsevier Science Publishing Company, Inc. from"Treatment Effects of Alprazolam and Imipramine: Physiological Versus Subjective Changes in Patients With Generalized Anxiety Disorder," by McLeod DR, Hoehn-Saric R, Zimmerli WD, et al. *Biological Psychiatry* 28:849–861, 1990. Copyright 1990 by the Society of Biological Psychiatry.

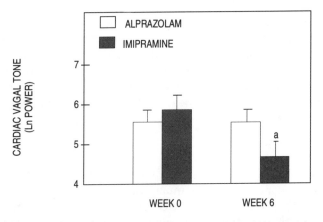

Figure 6–4. Six-week effects of alprazolam *(light histograms)* and imipramine *(dark histograms)* on cardiac vagal tone. a: Week 0 and Week 6 values differ ($P < .001$). Values represent the mean ±1 SE.

al. 1979), which represents the within-subject variance between individual heart interbeat intervals. As Figure 6–3 demonstrates, the within-subject variability in heart rate was decreased substantially by imipramine. This finding is consistent with the variability hypothesis. However, no decrease in variability occurred in the interbeat intervals of the alprazolam group despite the fact that this group also reported decreases in cardiovascular symptoms.

The second measure of heart rate variability consists of respiratory sinus arrhythmia, which is the variability in heart rate associated with respiration. A spectral analysis of the oscillations in heart rate was performed during periods of quiet rest. The power associated with the breathing frequencies represents respiratory sinus arrhythmia, which can be used as an index of cardiac vagal, or parasympathetic, tone (Porges 1986; Porges and Bohrer 1990). The effects of 6 weeks of medication on cardiac vagal tone are shown in Figure 6–4. Clearly, imipramine had a substantial decreasing effect on cardiac vagal tone, once again consistent with the variability hypothesis, whereas, inconsistent with the variability hypothesis, alprazolam had no effect at all.

The findings presented in Figures 6–3 and 6–4 demonstrate that although the variability hypothesis may account for some of the discrepancy between physiological measures and verbal report, other factors must also play a role. Moreover, because the alprazolam group reported decreased anxiety but no changes in heart rate variability, it is likely that the reduction in heart rate variability and cardiac vagal tone seen in the imipramine group was a direct effect of imipramine rather than an indirect effect of decreased anxiety.

Attention

Another possibility is that patients who have been treated for anxiety are just not paying as much attention to physiological changes as they were prior to treatment. This explanation is consistent with the attention hypothesis, which suggests that awareness of bodily states is greater with increased self-attention (Hansen et al. 1989; Scheier et al. 1983). Some support for the self-attention hypothesis comes from a study by Weisz et al. (1988), in which subjects performed heartbeat discrimination tasks more accurately when a mirror was placed in front of them.

Pennebaker (1982) has proposed a "competition of cues" hypothesis that states that awareness of internal stimuli is a function of the ratio of internal to external stimuli. According to this hypothesis, the more a person attends to external information, the less he or she will attend to internal information and the fewer (or milder) the symptoms he or she will report having. In addition, Pennebaker (in press) has provided evidence suggesting that men tend to rely more on internal stimuli, whereas women tend to rely more on external sources of information in the perception of bodily states. In a similar fashion, awareness of one physiological activity, such as heart rate, will depend on how much information is being processed from other physiological activities. In the present case, anxiety reduction could have resulted in more attention to external activities and less attention to internal sensations.

Expectation

The influence of expectations on subjective experience is well known. For example, van den Hout and Griez (1982) found that the effects of carbon dioxide inhalation depended on whether subjects were told to expect a state of pleasant relaxation or unpleasant feelings of tension. Similar results were reported by van der Molen et al. (1986) with subjects given sodium lactate infusions. Rapee et al. (1986) gave half of their panic disorder patients an explanation of the effects of carbon dioxide but gave the other half of their patients no explanation. Upon inhalation of carbon dioxide, the group who had not received an explanation reported marked panic symptoms, whereas the group who had received one reported only mild symptoms.

Expectations reflect a person's beliefs, and a person's beliefs can play a major role in determining his or her perceptions of physiological activity. A good example of this is found in a study by Pennebaker and Skelton (1981). Some subjects were told that an ultrasonic noise would increase skin temperature, while others were told that the noise would decrease skin temperature. After exposure to 2 minutes of silence, during which subjects believed they were being exposed to ultrasonic noise, subjects who were told that the procedure would increase skin temperature reported increases in finger temperature, while subjects who were told that the procedure would decrease skin temperature reported decreases in finger temperature. In reality, skin temperature neither increased nor decreased. Thus, perception of skin temperature was related not to actual skin temperature but to what subjects were told to believe. Other studies have produced similar results (Pennebaker and Epstein 1983).

Perhaps the apparent contradiction between the results of our earlier study, in which physiological and symptom report measures changed in the same direction under stress, and those of our more recent study, in which imipramine produced changes in physiological measures that were opposite those of the symptom reports, can be resolved by examining the expectations of the patients in the two studies. It seems reasonable to suppose that in the first study, patients expected increases under stress in heart rate and muscle tension, and reported as much. But it also seems reasonable to suppose that patients expected treatment to decrease heart rate and muscle tension, and that is what they reported in the second study. Unfortunately, expectations were neither measured nor manipulated in these studies. Future studies will be necessary to test this hypothesis.

CONCLUSIONS

It is unclear at the present time whether anxious patients are any more accurate in perceiving bodily states than nonanxious persons. Accuracy of physiological perception in patients with anxiety disorders is quite low when correlational analyses are used to measure it. By using categorical, rather than correlational, analysis, however, we have found that there are occasions in which patients can accurately perceive the direction, if not the degree, of change in physiological activities.

But there are also conditions in which anxiety patients report symptom changes that are inconsistent with those of the actual physiological referents. To determine the conditions under which patients will or will not accurately perceive physiological activity, we must first distinguish between detection and perception. Perception involves information from a variety of sources other than the physiological referent itself, and somatic symptom reports involve perception, not detection.

Three hypotheses—the variability hypothesis, the attention hypothesis, and the expectation hypothesis—are consistent with the findings of several studies on physiological perception. These hypotheses need to be tested further in future studies.

We began this chapter with a question: Should we believe our patients' somatic symptom reports? Unfortunately, the answer is not straightforward. It can be "yes" or "no" depending upon the context in which the question is asked. Therefore, when knowledge of physiological activity is important, actual physiological measures should be taken.

In summary, for both clinical and theoretical reasons, it is important to know how well patients can perceive bodily changes. For example, the choice of treatment regimens is often determined on the basis of somatic symptom reports. In this chapter we examined what is known about the relationship between somatic symptom reports and their underlying physiological referents in patients with anxiety disorders. While many studies have found low correlations between these two sets of measures, recent studies have shown that correlational analyses can be misleading. Results of studies using correlational analyses were compared with those of studies using categorical analyses, and the latter type of analysis was found to have certain advantages in cases where qualitative questions were posed. Also, a distinction was drawn between detection and perception, and the usefulness of this distinction in the study of somatic symptom reports was demonstrated. It was argued that somatic symptom reports reflect perception rather than detection, and theories of symptom perception that are consistent with the findings of recent studies—the variability hypothesis, the attention hypothesis, and the expectation hypothesis—were discussed. We concluded by suggesting that there are definitely circumstances in which patients with anxiety can accurately perceive the direction, if not the degree, of changes in physiological activities.

REFERENCES

Barlow DH, Mavissakalian MR, Schofield LD: Patterns of desynchrony in agoraphobia: a preliminary report. Behaviour Research and Therapy 18:441–448, 1980

Beck AT, Emery G: Anxiety Disorders and Phobias: A Cognitive Perspective. New York, Basic Books, 1985

Brener J, Kluvitse C: Heartbeat detection: judgments of the simultaneity of external stimuli and heartbeats. Psychophysiology 25:554–561, 1988

Clark DM: A cognitive approach to panic. Behaviour Research and Therapy 24:461–470, 1986

Ehlers A, Margraf J, Roth WT, et al: Anxiety induced by false heart rate feedback in patients with panic disorder. Behaviour Research and Therapy 26:1–11, 1988

Freedman RR, Ianni P, Ettedgui E, et al: Ambulatory monitoring of panic disorder. Arch Gen Psychiatry 42:244–248, 1985

Gaffney FA, Fenton BJ, Lane LD, et al: Hemodynamic, ventilatory, and biochemical responses of panic patients and normal controls with sodium lactate infusion and spontaneous panic attacks. Arch Gen Psychiatry 45:53–60, 1988

Grey S, Sartory G, Rachman S: Synchronous and desynchronous changes during fear reduction. Behaviour Research and Therapy 17:137–147, 1979

Hamilton M: The assessment of anxiety states by rating. Br J Med Psychol 32:50–55, 1959

Hansen RD, Hansen CH, Crano WD: Sympathetic arousal and self-attention: the accessibility of interoceptive and exteroceptive arousal cues. Journal of Experimental and Social Psychology 25:437–449, 1989

Heslegrave RJ, Ogilvie JC, Furedy JJ: Measuring baseline-treatment differences in heart rate variability: variance versus successive difference mean square and beats per minute versus interbeat interval. Psychophysiology 16:151–157, 1979

Hoehn-Saric R: Characteristics of chronic anxiety patients, in Anxiety: New Research and Changing Concepts. Edited by Klein DF, Rabkin JG. New York, Raven, 1981, pp 399–409

Hoehn-Saric R, McLeod DR, Zimmerli WD: Somatic manifestations in women with generalized anxiety disorder: psychophysiological responses to psychological stress. Arch Gen Psychiatry 46:1113–1119, 1989

Hoehn-Saric R, McLeod DR, Zimmerli WD: Psychophysiological response patterns in panic disorder. Acta Psychiatr Scand 83:4–11, 1991

Katkin ES: Blood, sweat and tears: individual differences in autonomic self-perception. Psychophysiology 22:125–137, 1985

Knight ML, Borden RJ: Autonomic and affective reactions of high and low socially-anxious individuals awaiting public performance. Psychophysiology 16:209–213, 1979

MacKay CJ: The measurement of mood and psychophysiological activity using self-report techniques, in Techniques in Psychophysiology. Edited by Martin I, Venables PH. New York, Wiley, 1980, pp 501–562

Margraf J, Taylor CB, Ehlers A, et al: Panic attacks in the natural environment. J Nerv Ment Dis 175:558–565, 1987

Mavissakalian M, Michelson L: Patterns of psychophysiological change in the treatment of agoraphobia. Behaviour Research and Therapy 20:347–356, 1982

McLeod DR, Hoehn-Saric R: Anxiety states, in Principles and Practice of Biological Psychiatry, Vol 2. Edited by Dinan TG. London, Clinical Neuroscience Publisher, 1990, pp 43–78

McLeod DR, Hoehn-Saric R, Stefan RL: Somatic symptoms of anxiety: comparison of self-report and physiological measures. Biol Psychiatry 21:301–310, 1986

McLeod DR, Hoehn-Saric R, Zimmerli WD, et al: Treatment effects of alprazolam and imipramine: physiological versus subjective changes in patients with generalized anxiety disorder. Biol Psychiatry 28:849–861, 1990

Montgomery WA, Jones GE: Laterality, emotionality, and heartbeat perception. Psychophysiology 21:459–465, 1984

Montgomery WA, Jones GE, Hollandsworth JG Jr: The effects of physical fitness and exercise on cardiac awareness. Biol Psychol 18:11–22, 1984

Morrow GR, Labrum AH: The relationship between psychological and physiological measures of anxiety. Psychol Med 8:95–101, 1978

Pennebaker JW: The Psychology of Physical Symptoms. New York, Springer, 1982

Pennebaker JW: Beyond laboratory-based cardiac perception: ecological interoception, in Advances in Cardiac Perception. Edited by Schandry R, Vaitl D. New York, Springer (in press)

Pennebaker JW, Epstein D: Implicit psychophysiology: effects of common beliefs and idiosyncratic physiological responses on symptom reporting. J Pers 51:468–496, 1983

Pennebaker JW, Hoover CW: Visceral perception versus visceral detection: disentangling methods and assumptions. Biofeedback Self Regul 9:339–352, 1984

Pennebaker JW, Skelton JA: Selective monitoring of physical sensations. J Pers Soc Psychol 41:213–223, 1981

Porges SW: Respiratory sinus arrhythmia: physiological basis, quantitative methods, and clinical implications, in Cardiorespiratory and Cardiosomatic Psychophysiology. Edited by Grossman P, Janssen KHL, Vaitl D. New York, Plenum, 1986, pp 101–115

Porges SW, Bohrer RE: The analysis of periodic processes in psychophysiological research, in Principles of Psychophysiology: Physical, Social, and Inferential Elements. Edited by Cacioppo JT, Tassinary LG. New York, Cambridge University Press, 1990, pp 708–753

Pyke RE, Greenberg HS: Norepinephrine challenges in panic patients. J Clin Psychopharmacol 6:279–285, 1986

Rachman S, Hodgson R: Synchrony and desynchrony in fear and avoidance. Behaviour Research and Therapy 12:311–318, 1974

Rapee R, Mattick R, Murrell E: Cognitive mediation in the affective component of spontaneous panic attacks. J Behav Ther Exp Psychiatry 17:245–253, 1986

Ray WJ, Cole HW, Raczynski JM: Psychophysiological assessment, in The Clinical Psychology Handbook. Edited by Hersen J, Kazdin AE, Bellack AS. New York, Pergamon, 1983, pp 427–453

Reed S, Harver A, Katkin E: Interoception, in Principles of Psychophysiology: Physical, Social, and Inferential Elements. Edited by Cacioppo JT, Tassinary LG. New York, Cambridge University Press, 1990, pp 253–291

Roth WT, Telch MJ, Taylor CB, et al: Autonomic changes after treatment of agoraphobia with panic attacks. Psychiatry Res 24:95–107, 1988

Sartory G, Rachman S, Grey S: An investigation of the relation between reported fear and heart rate. Behaviour Research and Therapy 15:435–438, 1977

Schandry R: Heartbeat perception and emotional experience. Psychophysiology 18:483–488, 1981

Schandry R, Specht G: The influence of psychological and physical stress on the perception of heartbeats (abstract). Psychophysiology 18:154, 1981

Scheier MF, Carver CS, Mathews KA: Attentional factors in the perception of bodily states, in Social Psychophysiology: A Sourcebook. Edited by Cacioppo JT, Petty RE. New York, Guilford, 1983, pp 510–542

Scott SB, Kessler M: An attempt to relate test anxiety and Palmer Sweat Index. Psychonomic Science 15:90–91, 1969

Sharpley CF, Fleming RK: Awareness of heart-rate reactivity. Psychol Rep 63:995–996, 1988

Skelton JA, Pennebaker JW: The verbal system, in Principles of Psychophysiology: Physical, Social, and Inferential Elements. Edited by Cacioppo JT, Tassinary LG. New York, Cambridge University Press, 1990, pp 631–657

Spielberger CS, Gorsuch RL, Lushene R: Manual for the State-Trait Anxiety Inventory. Palo Alto, CA, Consulting Psychologists Press, 1970

Stern R, Marks I: Brief and prolonged flooding: a comparison in agoraphobic patients. Arch Gen Psychiatry 28:270–276, 1973

Stroop JR: Interference in serial verbal reactions. Journal of Experimental Psychology 18:643–661, 1935

Taylor CB, Telch MJ, Havvik D: Ambulatory heart rate changes during panic attacks. J Psychiatr Res 17:261–266, 1983

Taylor CB, Sheikh J, Agras WS, et al: Ambulatory heart rate changes in patients with panic attacks. Am J Psychiatry 143:478–482, 1986

Thyer BA, Papsdorf JD, Davis R, et al: Autonomic correlates of the subjective anxiety scale. J Behav Ther Exp Psychiatry 15:3–7, 1984

Tyrer PJ, Lader MH: Central and peripheral correlates of anxiety: a comparative study. J Nerv Ment Dis 162:99–104, 1976

Tyrer P, Lee I, Alexander J: Awareness of cardiac function in anxious, phobic and hypochondriacal patients. Psychol Med 10:171–174, 1980

van den Hout MA, Griez E: Cognitive factors in carbon dioxide therapy. J Psychosom Res 26:209–214, 1982

van der Molen GM, van den Hout MA, Vroemen J, et al: Cognitive determinants of lactate-induced anxiety. Behaviour Research and Therapy 24:677–680, 1986

Vermilyea JA, Boice R, Barlow DH: Rachman and Hodgson (1974) a decade later: how do desynchronous response systems relate to the treatment of agoraphobia? Behaviour Research and Therapy 22:615–621, 1984

Weisz J, Balázs L, Adám G: The influence of self-focused attention on heartbeat perception. Psychophysiology 25:193–199, 1988

Whitehead WE, Drescher VM, Heiman P, et al: Relation of heart rate control to heartbeat perception. Biofeedback Self Regul 2:371–392, 1977

Zillmann D: Transfer of excitation in emotional behavior, in Social Psychophysiology: A Sourcebook. Edited by Cacioppo JT, Petty RE. New York, Guilford, 1983, pp 215–240

Chapter 7

Concluding Remarks

Rudolf Hoehn-Saric, M.D., and
Daniel R. McLeod, Ph.D.

Anxiety is a complex emotion in which heightened arousal, autonomic activation, the perception of physical changes, conditioned responses, cognitive elaborations, and decision making merge into a tapestry that can depict a simple fear response or an elaborate life-style. Obviously, no single system can be responsible for the biological manifestations of anxiety. It is necessary to see anxiety as the end product of interactions between several systems involving nuclei of the brain stem, the limbic system, and the prefrontal and temporal cortices. Various levels of interaction between these systems may shape individual experiences. Variations within the systems may also be responsible for the diversity of clinical manifestations seen in different anxiety disorders. It is not surprising, therefore, that research on anxiety gives rise to as many questions as it does answers.

Neuroimaging techniques will be particularly helpful in identifying areas of the brain associated with, and possibly responsible for, anxiety reactions. As Wilson and Mathew (Chapter 1) point out, equipment with better resolution, ligands identifying specific receptors, and techniques that permit studies of specific metabolic processes are currently being developed. Particularly useful will be the application of tracers with short half-lives that permit repeated imaging during the same session. These methods will permit us to examine several psychological and pharmacological interventions in sequence or to follow dynamic changes associated with any one intervention at given points in time.

Studies have already identified some areas of the brain associated with certain anxiety disorders, such as hyperfrontality in

245

obsessive-compulsive disorder (OCD), metabolic differences in the parahippocampal gyri in panic disorder, and increased perfusion of the temporal poles during anticipatory anxiety and sodium lactate–induced panic attacks. The causes of these changes are not known. They may represent areas of primary disturbances or secondary involvement. For instance, does the hyperfrontality of a patient with OCD mean that this disorder is a dysfunction of the prefrontal cortex and cingulate gyrus, or does it reflect, as some have speculated, a compensatory mechanism in response to a primary disturbance in the basal ganglia? Does anxiety increase or decrease cerebral blood flow? Studies suggest both. It appears that anxiety increases, but that concomitant hyperventilation decreases the cerebral blood flow. How do these two effects interact and what are the physiological and phenomenological results of this interaction? Many such questions should be answered in the near future.

Equally exciting are the advances made in our understanding of the role of neurotransmitters in anxiety. While discussing new research on the locus coeruleus–norepinephrine system at the meeting of the American College of Neuropsychopharmacology in December 1991, Floyd Bloom commented on how difficult it was to get grant support for studies of this system a decade ago. This was because granting agencies believed that the system was already well known and that not much new could be found. The presentations that Bloom discussed, however, were full of new findings, showing the intricacy and versatility of this apparently simple system. For instance, in monkeys, intermediate levels of activity in this system are associated with performance that is superior to that associated with either high or low levels of activity. This finding provided physiological confirmation of a phenomenon well known to psychologists since the early part of the century as the Yerkes-Dodson Law. That is, best performance is associated with moderate levels of arousal and becomes poorer in a state of low or high arousal. Thus, even the apparently well-explored role of the noradrenergic system in the biology of anxiety remains a source of new discoveries.

Kahn and Moore's survey of the serotonergic system in anxiety (see Chapter 2) describes how important, but also how complicated, the system really is. Recent studies show convincingly that alterations in serotonin levels affect panic attacks, directly or possibly indirectly, as well as psychological components of anxiety. The mechanisms of action are still unclear because the serotonergic receptor system is far more complex than that of the noradrenergic system and sufficient receptor-specific agonists and antagonists are not presently available for human studies. We do know, however, that stimulation of the serotonin 5-HT$_{1A}$ receptor and the blockade of the 5-HT$_2$ receptor produce anxiolytic effects in generalized anxiety but are ineffective in the prevention of panic attacks. We also know that stimulation of the 5-HT$_{1C}$ and 5-HT$_3$ receptors produces anxiety. Thus, anxiety is not induced or reduced simply by either a deficiency or an excess of serotonin in the brain, but rather by changes affecting delicate balances within the serotonergic system that are, to a large extent, still unknown. In their survey, Kahn and Moore formulated a plausible theory of the pathology of the serotonergic system in anxiety based on Kahn's and his colleagues' research.

Another rapidly advancing area of research involves neuropeptides. A constantly increasing number of neuropeptides that act as neurotransmitters or modulators are being identified. Some neuropeptides actually coexist with classical neurotransmitters in the same brain cells. Thus, the presence of neuropeptides may be responsible for the differential effects of neurotransmitters in certain regions of the brain. Several neuropeptides have been found to induce anxiety in animals or humans, but the best researched neuropeptide, associated with anxiety as well as depression, is corticotropin-releasing factor (CRF). As reviewed by Pihoker and Nemeroff in Chapter 3, CRF not only causes the same physiological and behavioral changes in animals that occur naturally during stress, but affects the same brain-stem nuclei and limbic lobe structures that are associated with anxiety. Moreover, anxiety is frequently present in depression, and many "pure" anxiety patients, at some stage, develop depression. A disturbance of the CRF system, which is disturbed in both anxiety and depression, may be a reason that anxiety and depression frequently coexist. Undoubtedly, research will uncover other neuropeptides closely linked to anxiety.

When we become anxious we tend to associate the situation in which we have become anxious with the anxiety we experience.

Thus, a learning process takes place. The learning of cues that we associate with potential harm forms the basis for the cognitive-affective warning system that is essential for our survival. The research of Post and his colleagues, described in Chapter 4, addressed two issues: 1) the mechanisms that make such learning possible and 2) anomalies of the same processes that lead to kindling and possibly to the development of panic disorder. Both processes require the induction of long-term potentiation in neurons of the hippocampus and possibly other parts of the limbic system, as well as the activation of the third-messenger system for their fixation. Both processes are modified through input from the noradrenergic, serotonergic, and GABAergic systems, as well as from CRF. Work by Post and others will continue to shed light on the interactions between anxiety, learning (including the acquisition of phobias), and kindling processes, which are possibly responsible for the paroxysmal nature of some anxiety disorders.

Anxiety always has been associated with symptoms suggesting muscular and autonomic activation. In Chapter 5, on somatic manifestations of normal and pathological anxiety, Hoehn-Saric and McLeod described recent studies demonstrating that physiological responses associated with anxiety differ among patients with different anxiety disorders as well as between patients having the same anxiety disorder. Interestingly, diminished autonomic flexibility was found in all examined anxiety disorders. It will be interesting to see whether this decreased autonomic flexibility is specific for anxiety disorders or if it can occur in other psychiatric disorders as well. Presently we do not know if this phenomenon is the result of excessive preoccupation with potential danger or physical discomfort leading to inattention to cues and interactions that do not appear to be related to the source of anxiety, an adaptation to the physiological stress of chronic anxiety, or a trait marker. Advanced techniques that measure sympathetic and parasympathetic activity, ambulatory monitor studies that record autonomic states in real-life situations, neurohumoral measures, psychological and pharmacological challenges, imaging studies that relate peripheral with central phenomena, and family and genetic studies promise to shed new light on the still baffling differences in physiological responses.

It is important to know how well patients with anxiety can perceive bodily changes and give accurate somatic symptom reports. But although relationships between the subjective and physiological have long been the subject of intense research, conclusions reached only a few short years ago are currently being challenged. This is because our conclusions have been determined in large part by our procedures and methods of analysis. In Chapter 6, on the perception of physiological changes in normal and pathological anxiety, McLeod and Hoehn-Saric pointed out the need to examine not only the physiological activities themselves but the role of other factors that contribute to somatic symptom reports.

This book is not a comprehensive review of recent advancements in our understanding of the biology of anxiety. For lack of space many fields of research in anxiety had to be omitted. The areas presented, however, represent some of the most exciting developments in the field. Our knowledge of anxiety is like a partially filled puzzle that permits only the recognition of vague shapes and outlines. Hopefully the chapters in this book will help to make the picture of the puzzle a bit more recognizable.

Index

*Note: Page numbers printed in **boldface** type refer to tables or figures.*

Acetazolamide, **33**, 37–38
ACTH (adrenocorticotropin), 105–106
Adaptation, chronic stress, 184, 193
Adinazolam, 112–113
Adrenocorticotropin. *See* ACTH
Affective disorders
  ACTH response to CRF, 114
  contingent tolerance, 163
  procaine and mood changes, 129
Aggression, 90
Agoraphobia
  heart rate and desynchrony, 231–232
  imipramine and, 127
  panic disorder and serotonin, 74
  physiological responses to behavioral interactions, 203
Alcohol, 165
Alprazolam
  cocaine-induced panic attacks, 127, 149
  corticotropin-releasing factor and, 112–113
  patient perception of physiological symptoms, 230–232, 233–237
Amphetamines, 129
Amygdala-kindled seizures
  c-fos induction, 145–146, 157
  effects of carbamazepine on, 122, 135, 161–163
Anesthetics, local, 131–134

Animals
  phobia of and CBF levels, 41
  studies of serotonin and anxiety, 63–71, **72–73**
Anorexia nervosa, 114
Anticipatory anxiety, 23, 45
Anxiety. *See also specific disorders;* Stress
  activation of autonomic nervous system, 17
  arousal and relationship to, 10
  blood viscosity and CBF, 18
  carbon dioxide levels, 19–20
  cerebral blood flow (CBF)
    CMR under resting conditions and, 24–29
    factors influencing relationship with, 43–45
    future directions of research on, 46–47
    induction and changes in, 32–43
    regional values and ratings of, 24
    study of and, 9
    variables influencing, **14**
  cocaine-related panic reactions, 129
  corticotropin-releasing factor (CRF)
    anxiogenic effects and, 107–108, 110
    anxiolytics and, 111–13
    in patients with anxiety disorders, 114–115
  electrical stimulation, 132

Anxiety *(continued)*
  epinephrine and norepinephrine
    in periphery, 15
  normal as biological warning
    system, 177
  perception of physiological
    changes in
    accuracy of self-reports,
      223–224
    correlational versus
      categorical analysis,
      229–230
    correlations between
      symptom reports and
      physiology, 226–227
    desynchrony and, 230–232
    detection compared with,
      232–233
    mechanisms of, 233–237
    symptoms and, 224–226
  pulse rate and elevation of
    blood pressure, 20
  serotonin
    animal experiments and,
      63–71
    future research on role in,
      89–91
    studies of role in human,
      71–89
    studies of role in
      pathogenesis of, 61
  somatic manifestations
    diminished autonomic
      flexibility, 207–209
    measurement, 177–179
    summary of, 209–211
    stress and relationship to,
      20–21, 103–104
Apprehension, 23
Arousal
  accuracy in visceral perception,
    224–225
  anxiety and relationship to, 10

brain-stem reticular formation
    and, 2
  cerebral blood flow (CBF)
    brain stem and CMR levels,
      12, 43
    frontal cortex and, 12–13, 43
    global changes in CMR and,
      11
    hyperfrontal pattern of
      distribution, 8, 43
  cerebral cortex and, 2–4
  definition of concept, 1
  frontal lobes and, 8
  limbic system and, 2
  simple phobias and autonomic,
    186
Arrhythmias, 205, 235
Atropine, **138**
Attention hypothesis, 236
Autonomic nervous system
  CBF and acute anxiety, 17
  role of in initiation of panic
    attacks, 204

Behavior, anxiogenic, 108, 110
Behavioral interactions, 203
Behavioral sensitization, 123,
    129–31
Behavioral stimulation, **33**
ß-Endorphin, 159
Benzodiazepines
  anxiogenic behavior and CRF,
    108, 110
  cocaine-induced panic attacks,
    135, 139
  contingent-tolerance
    mechanisms, 122, 164–165
  effect on CRF concentration in
    brain, 114–115
  GAD patients and CMR, 42
  lidocaine-kindled seizures,
    134–135

Blood-injury phobias, 187–188, 210

Blood pressure, 184, 187, 188

Blood viscosity, 18

Borderline personality disorder, 129

Bradycardia, 187, 188

Brain. *See also* Cerebral blood flow (CBF); Cerebral metabolic rate (CMR)
anatomy and physiology of serotonin in, 61–63
neurophysiology of arousal and anxiety, 1–4
research on abnormal function in psychiatric disorders, 10
structure and activity of CRF, 105

Brain hemispheres, 3–4

Brain stem, 12

Brain-stem reticular formation, 2

Buspirone, 78, 87–88

Caffeine
anxiety induction and CBF/ CMR changes, 32, **33**, 34–35
c-fos induction, 146–150
panic patients and effects and/or avoidance of, 154

Carbamazepine
amygdala-kindled seizures, 122, **138**, 161–163
chronic and cocaine-kindled seizures and deaths, **137**
cocaine-related panic attacks, 127, 139
contingent tolerance, 165
cross-tolerance for benzodiazepine ligands, **164**
lidocaine- and cocaine-induced kindled seizures, 125, 135, **136**

local-anesthetic–kindled seizures, 141

Carbon dioxide
anxiety and CBF/CMR levels, 19–20, **33**, 36–37, 46
expectations and physiological response, 236–237

Cardiovascular disease, 205, 211

Cardiovascular system. *See* Cardiovascular disease; Heart rate

Catecholamines
anxiety and changes in CBF and CMR, 15–16
cocaine and acute mechanisms, 127–129
diminished autonomic flexibility, 207–208
gender and acute stress response, 181, 182

Categorical analysis, 229–230

Central nervous system (CNS)
heterogeneous distribution of CRF, 107
serotonin receptors, 62–63

Cerebral autoregulation, 20

Cerebral blood flow (CBF)
anxiety induction, 32–43
autonomic nervous system and, 17
brain stem and activity, 12
carbon dioxide levels, 19–20
catecholamines and, 15–16
factors influencing relationship with anxiety, 43–45
frontal cortex and arousal, 12–13
future directions of research, 46–47
gender and, 20
global changes in and arousal, 11
hemorheology and, 17–19

Cerebral blood flow *(continued)*
  hyperfrontality and, 7–10
  measurement techniques and
      issues, 4–7
  pulse rate and perfusion
      pressure, 20
  resting conditions, 24–29
  stress and, 21–24
  tranquilization and, 13–14
  variables influencing, **14**
Cerebral cortex, 2–4
Cerebral ischemia, 45
Cerebral metabolic rate (CMR)
  anxiety induction and, 32–43
  brain stem and activity, 12
  carbon dioxide levels, 19
  catecholamines and, 15
  factors influencing relationship
      with anxiety, 43–45
  future directions of research,
      46–47
  gender and, 20
  global changes in and arousal,
      11
  measurement techniques and
      issues, 4–7
  obsessive-compulsive disorder
      (OCD), 29–32
  resting conditions, 24–29
  stress and, 21–24
  variables influencing, **14**
Cerebral vasoconstriction, 35,
      41–42
Challenge paradigm, 74
Checking behavior, 207
Children
  early stress, trauma, or
      maternal neglect and
      affective and/or anxiety
      disorders in adulthood, 113
  PET study of onset of
      obsessive-compulsive
      disorder (OCD), 31

Chlordiazepoxide, 108, **109**
p-Chlorophenylalanine (p-CPA),
      64, **65**, 66
m-Chlorophenylpiperazine
      (m-CPP)
  c-fos induction, 153–154
  serotonin and panic disorders,
      79–81, 83, 89
Cholecystokinin, 153–154
Cinanserin, 67
Clomipramine
  obsessive-compulsive disorder
      (OCD)
    and CMR levels, 31
    and serotonin, 82, 83, 87
  panic disorder and serotonin,
      74–75
Clonidine, **138**
Cocaine
  c-fos induction, 150
  clinical implications of studies,
      121–122
  kindling of panic disorder,
      122–141
  panic disorder related to,
      125–127
Comatose states, 12
Competition of cues hypothesis,
      236
Computed tomography (CT)
      scanning, 9
Conditioned avoidance learning,
      157159
Conditioned emotional response
      (CER) model, 63
Conditioning, cocaine-induced
      behavioral sensitization, 123
Conflict paradigm, 63
Correlational analysis, 229–230
Corticotropin-releasing factor
      (CRF)
  anxiogenic effects, 107–108, 110
  anxiolytics and, 111–113

c-fos induction, **158**
cocaine and release of, 141
effects of stress on, 110–111
localization of, 106–107
in patients with anxiety
    disorders, 114–115
structure and activity of,
    104–106
Cortisol
acute stress response, 181
adaptation to chronic stress, 184
obsessive-compulsive disorder
    (OCD), 207
response to m-CPP, 80
simple phobias, 185–186
Cyproheptadine, 67, 70

Depression
cocaine-related panic, 129
cortisol nonsuppression after
    dexamethasone
    administration, 114
hyperactivity of CRF neurons,
    114
obsessive-compulsive disorder
    (OCD) and CMR levels,
    29–30
as result of stress from
    pathological anxiety, 104
serotonin and anxiety, 88, 90
Desipramine (DMI), **140**
Desynchrony, 230–232
Diazepam
amygdala-kindled seizures,
    135, **138**
contingent tolerance, 163–164
generalized anxiety disorder
    (GAD) and serotonin, 88
hyperfrontality and CBF
    distribution, 8
tranquilization and CBF,
    13–14

Dihydroxytryptamine (DHT),
    66–67
Diminished autonomic flexibility,
    207–209, 211
Direct variability hypothesis, 234
Doom anxiety, 131
Dopamine, 127–128
Dreaming, 11

Electrical stimulation, 132
Electroconvulsive seizure (ECS),
    143–145
Electrodermal activity, **200**
Electroencephalogram (EEG), 11
Electroencephalography, 10
Emotions
animal laboratory studies of
    anxiety, 63–64
subjective experiences of and
    neurobiological
    differences, 10
Epilepsy, 163
Epinephrine
acute stress response, 181
anxiety induction and CBF, **33**,
    35–36
CBF and cerebral metabolism,
    15–16, 43
stress and increased CBF, 21
Esophagospasms, 183
Expectation hypothesis, 236–237

Family history, 183
Fenfluramine, 80, 89
FG 7142, 152
Fluoxetine, 75, 83
Fluvoxamine, 75, 78, 82
Fos-Jun complex, 155
Frontal cortex, 12–13
Frontal lobes
arousal and association with, 8,
    43

Frontal lobes *(continued)*
  cerebral cortex and arousal, 2–3
  wakefulness and increased
    activity in, 7–8

Gamma-aminobutyric acid
    (GABA) complex, 90
Gender
  acute stress response and,
    181–182
  CBF and CMR levels, 20
  incidence of stress polycytosis,
    18
Generalized anxiety disorder
    (GAD)
  anxiety levels and CBF/CMR,
    44
  benzodiazepines and CMR, 42
  caffeine and CBF, 34
  carbon dioxide inhalation and
    anxiety induction, 36–37
  diminished autonomic
    flexibility, 208
  patient symptom reports,
    226–227
  somatic manifestations of
    anxiety, 194–196, 210
  stress and polycytosis, 18–19
  studies of anxiety and
    serotonin, 87–88, 89–90
Growth hormone, 181

Heart rate. *See also*
    Cardiovascular disease
  agoraphobia and imipramine,
    231–232
  blood-injury phobias, 187, 188
  panic attacks, 202–203, 229–230
  physiological measure in panic
    disorder patients, **198–199**
  social phobias, 189, 190

symptom perception, 225–226,
    233–237
Hematocrit, 17–18
Hemispheres, brain, 3–4
Hemorheology, 17–19
Heroin, 128
Hormonal response
  acute stress and, 181, 211
  generalized anxiety disorder
    (GAD), 195–196
  m-CPP, 80–81, 89
  panic disorders and, **200–201**,
    205
  posttraumatic stress disorder
    (PTSD), 193
  simple phobias, 185–186
  social phobias, 189–190
Hotlines, cocaine, 123, 134
5-Hydroxyindoleacetic acid
    (5-HIAA), 71, 74
5-Hydroxytryptamine (5-HT). *See*
    Serotonin
Hyperfrontality, 7–10, 12–13, 43
Hyperventilation, 20, 180, 204–205
Hypocapnia, 20, 180
Hypothalamo-pituitary-adreno-
    cortical (HPA) axis, 105–106

Imipramine
  caffeine-induced panic attacks,
    149
  cocaine-related panic attacks,
    139
  patient perceptions of
    physiological symptoms of
    anxiety, 230–232, 233–237
  serotonin and panic disorders,
    74, 75, 78
Immediate-early genes, 143
Indirect variability hypothesis,
    234
Inner ear problems, 205

Interleukin-1, 159
Intracarotid inhalation and injection techniques, 4, **5**
Irritable bowel syndrome, 183
Ischemia, 205
Isoproterenol, 15–16, 153–154

James-Lange theory, 183

Kindling. *See also* Amygdala-kindled seizures; Cocaine
  implications of model for pharmacotherapeutics, 160–165
  phases of evolution, **124**

Lactate infusion, 44, 153–154. *See also* Sodium lactate
Learning, 157–159, 160
Left hemisphere, 3–4
Lidocaine, 124, 134–135
Limbic system, 2
Local-anesthetic–kindled seizures, 141
Locus coeruleus, 110
Long-term potentiation, 160
Lorazepam, 88

Maprotiline, 75
Marijuana, **33**, 38–39
Maternal neglect, 113
Mean square successive difference statistic (MSSD), 234–235
Memory, 159
Mental activity, 23
Metergoline, 67, 70
Methysergide, 67, 70
Mitral valve prolapse, 183, 205
MK 801, **138**
Muscular activity, 178–179, **200**, 210

Nitrous oxide inhalation technique, 4, **5**
Norepinephrine, 15, 16, 181
Novel environment model, 63–64

Obsessive-compulsive disorder (OCD)
  abnormal dopaminergic function, 90
  anxiety and CBF changes, 40–41
  CMR levels and, 29–32, 44
  diminished autonomic flexibility, 208
  somatic manifestations of anxiety, 205–207, 210
  studies of anxiety and serotonin, 81–87, 88–89, 89–90
Panic disorder
  ACTH response to CRF, 114
  caffeine and CBF, 34
  cocaine and clinical implications of studies, 121–122
  diminished autonomic flexibility, 208
  heart rate perception and, 229–230
  increased noradrenergic function as pathogenic factor, 90
  kindling of cocaine-related, 122–141
  lactate infusion and CBF, 40, 44
  neural substrates of panicogenic agents and proto-oncogene *c-fos*, 142–160
  patient symptom perception, 225
  serotonin and anxiety, 74–81, 88–89, 89–90

Panic disorder *(continued)*
   somatic manifestations of
      anxiety, 183–184, 196–205,
      210–211
   temporal lobe abnormalities, 3
   yohimbine and anxiety levels,
      40
Panicogenic agents, **133**, 142–160.
   See also specific medications
Patients, anxiety disorders
   accuracy of somatic symptom
      reports, 223–224
   correlational versus categorical
      analysis, 229–230
   correlations between symptom
      reports and physiology,
      226–227
   desynchrony and, 230–232
   mechanisms of symptom
      perception, 233–237
   perception of symptoms versus
      detection, 232–233
   symptom perception and
      anxiety, 224–226
Pentylenetetrazole, 128, 129,
   151–152
Perfusion pressure, 20
Personality, 181–182
Phenytoin, 135, **138**
Pheochromocytoma, 183
Phobias
   animal phobias and CBF levels,
      41
   diminished autonomic
      flexibility, 208
   physiological changes in anxiety
      disorders, 185–190, 210
PK 11195, 163
Polycytosis, 17–19
Positron-emission tomography
   (PET)
   CBF and CMR measurement
      techniques, 4, **5**, 6

global CMR and arousal, 11
hyperfrontality and glucose
   metabolism, 8
Posttraumatic stress disorder
   (PTSD)
   ACTH response to CRF, 114
   diminished autonomic
      flexibility, 208, 209
   somatic manifestations of
      anxiety, 191–194, 210
Prefrontal cortex, 127–128
Problem-solving tests, 12–13
Procaine, 129, 133
Prolactin, 181
Proto-oncogene *c-fos*, 142–160
Public speaking, 189
Pulse rate, 20

Rape victims, 193
Respiratory sinus arrhythmia, 235
Respiratory system, panic
   disorders and, **199–200**
Resting conditions, CBF levels
   and, 24–29, 44
Reticular neurons, 2
Right hemisphere, 3
Ritanserin
   generalized anxiety disorder
      (GAD) and, 87, 88
   serotonin and anxiety
      reduction, 67, 78

Seizures. *See* Amygdala-kindled
   seizures; Cocaine;
   Electroconvulsive seizures;
   Local-anesthetic–kindled
   seizures
Self-reports, 223–224
Serotonin (5-hydroxytryptamine
   [5-HT])
   anatomy and physiology in
      brain, 61–63

future research questions, 89–91
studies of anxiety in animals,
  63–71, **72–73**
studies of anxiety in humans,
  71–89
studies on role in pathogenesis
  of anxiety, 61
Sertraline, 82
Simple phobias, 185–186, 210
Single-photon emission
  computed tomography
  (SPECT), 4, **5**, 9
Skin conductance, 179, 185
Slow-wave sleep, 11
Social interaction model, 70–71
Social phobias, 188–190, 210
Sodium lactate, **33**, 39–40, 237. *See
  also* Lactate infusion
Somatic Symptoms Scale, 230
State-Trait Anxiety Inventory, 224
Stress. *See also* Anxiety
  acute psychophysiological
    effects of, 179–184
  anxiety induction and CBF, 42
  c-fos induction, 143–145
  cocaine and locomotor activity,
    141
  corticotropin-releasing factor
    and, 110–111
  definition of concept, 20–21
  epinephrine and norepinephrine
    in periphery, 15
  and pathological anxiety states,
    103–104
  somatic symptoms of anxiety,
    228
Stress polycytosis, 18–19
Stroop test, 226–227
Suicidal behavior, 90
Sweat glands, 179
Sympathetic fibers, 17
Sympathetic nervous system,
  sweat gland activity, 179

Tachyphylaxis, 131
Task administration, 23
Temporal lobes, 3
Three Mile Island nuclear
  accident, 184
Tolerance, contingent, 161–165
Tomography, 4, 7
Tracer-kinetic models, 6
Transcription factors, 142–143,
  155–160
Tranquilization, 13–14. *See also*
  specific medications
Trauma, childhood, 113
Trazodone, 30, 75
Triazolobenzodiazepines, 112–113
Tricyclic antidepressants, 82–83,
  139
Trigeminal neuralgia, 163, 165

Variability hypothesis, 233–236

Wakefulness, 3, 7–8
Water-lick model, 66
War veterans, 191–192, 194, 210

Xenon inhalation techniques, 6
X-maze anxiety model
  destruction of serotonin
    neurons, 66
  increase of serotonin function,
    70, 71
  methodological issues, 64

Yohimbine
  c-fos induction, 152–153
  panic disorders and CBF levels,
    39–40, 44
  physiological responses to
    panic attacks, 204

Zif/268, 159
Zimelidine, 75